Ready, Now

Your Guide to Doing Recovery from
Anorexia Nervosa Different this Time

By Bonnie Killip

A passionate and lavishly energetic biomedical scientist, health, and nutrition expert (APD), clinical and medical hypnotherapist, life and success coach, and ocean lover from the east coast of Australia, Bonnie Killip offers a whole new way of thinking about eating disorders.

In *Ready, Now,* Bonnie provides honest, practical, science backed, and at times challenging advice and insight into living with and recovering from anorexia nervosa that may change your life or the life of someone you love.

With my whole heart, these words are dedicated to those yet to come to know and love themselves.

Contents

Part One *Introduction*	**8**
1.1 Welcome to *Ready, Now*	9
1.2 Overview of Anorexia Nervosa	16
What is Anorexia Nervosa?	16
Core Psychopathology: Misidentification of Food as a Threat	17
Why do Some People Develop Anorexia Nervosa?	20
Summary to Overview of Anorexia Nervosa	23
Part Two *Psychological and Physiological Aspects of Anorexia Nervosa*	**24**
2.1 The Psychology of Anorexia Nervosa	24
Introduction to the Psychological Aspects of Anorexia Nervosa	25
Illness Process – Inside the Mind	25
Two Stages of the Illness Process	26
1. The Early Stages – Possessed	27
2. In the Depths of the Illness – Insight but Inability to Change	42
Conclusion to the Psychology of Anorexia Nervosa	50
2.2 The Physiology of Anorexia Nervosa	50
Introduction to the Physiology of Anorexia Nervosa	51
Starvation and Malnutrition	52
Metabolic Changes	54
Fat & Muscle Wastage	55
Normal Metabolism	55
Electrolyte Imbalances	58
Bones & Teeth	59
Hair, Nails, and Skin	60
Hormones and Menstruation	61
Emotions and Mood	65

Brain Changes	67
Lethargy, Headaches, Dizziness, and Fainting	68
Sleep Disturbances and Insomnia	69
Water Retention	70
Digestive Problems	71
Cholesterol Disturbances	72
Conclusion to the Physiological Aspects of Anorexia Nervosa	73
Part Three *Recovery*	**75**
3.1 An Introduction to Recovery	75
Recovery Disclaimer	76
What is Recovered?	83
How Do I Know When I am Recovered?	88
What is Recovery?	88
How Long Does Recovery Take?	90
3.2 Introduction to the Two Major Stages of Recovery	92
Introduction to The Two-Stages Model of Recovery	92
Stage One of Recovery: Surrender	93
Component One. Weight Gain	96
Introduction to Weight Gain	97
Component Two. Repair of Physical Damage	107
Introduction to Repair of Physical Damage	107
Refeeding & Refeeding Syndrome	111
Extreme Hunger (Hypermetabolism)	113
Night Sweats	118
Low Blood Glucose	119
Excessive Exercise	120
Digestive Problems	123
Exhaustion & Irritability	126
Micronutrient Deficiencies	128

Conclusion to Stage One: Surrender - Weight Gain and Repair of Physical Damage   129

   Stage Two of Recovery: Growth   130

   Component Three - Psychological Development   130

   Introduction to Psychological Development   130

   What is Psychological Development?   133

  3.3   Introducing the 6 Areas of Psychological Development   143

    1.   Welcome It   144

    2.   Decide   146

    3.   Know What You Want (Discovering and Living to Your Values)   151

    4.   Creating Empowering Beliefs   156

    5.   Developing your Capable Self-Identity   162

    6.   Giving Yourself Unconditional Permission   167

Conclusion to Psychological Development   170

   You are Not to Blame   171

Part Four *Treatment*   172

  4.1   Introduction to Treatment   172

   Defining Treatment   173

   What Do I Look for When Choosing Treatment?   175

   A Note on Current Treatment   179

   A Better Way   184

   Who Makes Up My Power Recovery Team?   188

  4.2   Introducing the Power Recovery Team   189

   1. Dietitian   192

   2. Clinical Hypnotherapist and Neurolinguistic Programming Practitioner   199

   3. Life Coach   213

   Summary to Recruiting Your Power Team   216

   What Matters Most When Choosing Help   216

   The Three Most Important Characteristics of Your Chosen Recovery Team   218

4.3	Environment	220
4.4	Into the World: Practice	220

Conclusion to *Ready, Now*   222

    5.1   Parting Words   226

Reference   228

Part One
Introduction

May every sunrise hold more promise and every sunset hold more peace.
~ Umair Siddiqui.

Hi, my name is Bonnie. I am a health and nutrition professional and founder and owner of Fuelling Success an Eating Disorder Recovery Consulting Service which facilitates people living with eating disorders to break free and live the rest of their lives in a different way.

My choice of profession was not random. I have lived two vastly different lives in relation to eating disorders.

I have also been the desperate, trapped, and confused patient in the hospital bed. This is why I now do the work I do. Because I know that no matter where you've been or where you are now, change is possible.

This is also why I was inspired to create *Ready, Now*.

Ready, Now was born from the combination of unspeakable heartbreak and a richness I could have gained by no other means than having lived on both sides of the hospital bed.

Ready, Now is my means of offering the answers to those questions I asked and had no answers for during what turned into fifteen years of relentless fighting, fear, uncertainty, cycles of giving in and giving up when I thought I could take no more, endless threats, and harsh attempts at self-motivating, intermingled with fleeting glimpses of excitement, joy, and hope. All bathed in the one thing that was constant and certain—the all-consuming shame as I tried to recover from an illness that dominated my existence. An illness I was repeatedly told there was no cure for and that I would either die from or have to manage for the rest of my life.

To say I know life with anorexia nervosa painfully well is an understatement. What is more important is that I also know life on the other side.

I know what is possible. I want you to know this too. I want you to not only hope and dream for a better future but to actually reach and live that better future.

1.1 Welcome to *Ready, Now*

Yesterday I was clever, so I wanted to change the world.
Today I am wise, so I am changing myself.
~ Rumi

If you have picked up this book, chances are high you have some understanding of what an eating disorder (ED) is, either because you or someone you care about is living with one.

Which means what you have also likely come to realise is that recovery from an ED requires more than having an understanding of what an ED is. For, no matter how great your understanding, whether it is you or a loved one who is living with an eating disorder, there are likely times you feel lost, angry, frustrated, overwhelmed, helpless, or hopeless with how to cope, let alone how to move forward.

I wrote *Ready, Now* first and foremost for those searching for the elusive and, in moments of utter despair, seemingly impossible pieces that occur between sick and recovered or what is commonly referred to as *recovery*.

I would also love for those helping a loved one through recovery or anyone who works in healthcare with people during their recoveries from EDs to choose to read *Ready, Now*.

Why? Because EDs are incredibly misunderstood illnesses, and gaining a deeper insight into the illness will give you the ability to help where others cannot. The value of which cannot be overstated.

For the most part, I will discuss in these pages the eating disorder diagnosis of anorexia nervosa, because this is the illness I am most intimately familiar with. However, there are similarities between EDs, especially in terms of the initiating and perpetuating factors as well as the key components of psychological recovery, development, and creating a new life. Which is why this book can be of great benefit to those recovering from, helping others recover from, or working with those in recovery from any of the many manifestations EDs come in.

Ready, Now is Unapologetically Life Focused

Complex does not mean impossible.
~ Bonnie Killip

If you were hoping for a romanticised or glamourous portrayal of anorexia nervosa or shocking skeletal "before" photos juxtaposed against plump, smiling "after" photos, you won't find it within these pages.

I wrote *Ready, Now* not to glorify my journey, nor simply to describe what an ED is, not to speculate on reasons as to why you may have developed one, nor to talk about how hard it is to live with an ED, not to help you feel momentarily supported, justified, or comfortable in the illness but rather as a frank and straightforward communication of the unwatered-down reality of living with and, most importantly, recovering from an ED.

I was called to create *Ready, Now* as a means of offering those who are interested in the practicalities of recovery—in other words; the "how to" behind what it takes to truly recover—my insight. Because when I was sick and seeking guidance, direction, and any semblance of certainty, they were nowhere to be found.

It is my intention, even though our journeys are different, that *Ready, Now* offers you a source of clarity amongst what can otherwise feel like horizonless chaos.

The Real Before and After

> *Your past is your unique collection of resources.*
> *~ Bonnie Killip.*

EDs are deeply cloaked in shame and misunderstanding.

An incredibly valuable experience during my recovery was to hear the stories of others who had gone through similar experiences to myself and fully recovered. Their stories reassured me that I wasn't alone in my "craziness". They let me know that maybe, just maybe, recovery was possible.

Therefore, although *Ready, Now* is by no stretch purely a recount of my story, throughout the following pages I do interweave a few of my experiences, thoughts, and insights with the intention that they spark within you the beginnings of self-compassion. I also do this to highlight the vast level of change between my past life with AN and my current life without AN because no matter how crazy, broken, beyond help, or unworthy of help you may now deem yourself, the truth is you are capable of monumental transformation. You are capable of a level of change and a new life that is so vastly different from what you are experiencing now, have ever experienced, or that you are likely able to yet imagine.

This is the real before and after.

Comfort is Not Synonymous with Cure

In any given moment, we have two options: to step forward into growth or to step back into safety.
~ Abraham Maslow.

Part of my motivation for writing this book was my desire to minimize your anxiety as you venture further from the monotonous, regimented, and often terrifyingly dangerous routine of anorexia and into completely uncharted territory. However, in no way does this mean this book is intended to placate or remove all your fear. In fact, I am confident you will find more than a few parts of this book confronting and uncomfortable, and I am happy knowing this. If I were to write a book solely to provide support and comfort, such a book, no matter how lovely and how pure the intentions, would not be serving you, because comfort is not synonymous with cure.

Your Fears Are Valid

Don't measure your progress using someone else's ruler.
~ Alessandra Olanow

There are no guarantees in recovery, just the same as there are no guarantees in life, which means your fears about the unknowns and struggles yet to come are valid.

However, the difference is, when you are recovered, all the unknowns and struggles are no longer cause for overwhelm and self-destruction, because it is you who is now better equipped to live and sometimes even learn and grow through them.

The struggles will come, the bad days will come, but, ultimately, the goal of recovery is that you change, and this new version of you will get through without self-abandonment.

Importantly, your change must be unconditional, and not dependant on anyone or anything else in the world changing with you.

Rather than leave this change up to chance, *Ready Now* is my contribution to introducing you to resources and tools that you may not have considered, understood, or even knew existed. I offer practical resources which are available to assist you in making real and profound change within your body, mind, and life.

A Fulfilling Life by Any Definition

Being free of the "problem" may be your highest dream of what is possible now, but one day you will look back and know it was just the beginning.
~ Bonnie Killip

I have a very strong definition of recovered, and it is distinct from the management or even the absence of the ED. My view of recovered is a life in which it no longer requires an internal battle to care for yourself because you now care for, love, and respect yourself naturally, easily, and effortlessly. Surely, the goal of not only recovery but a fulfilling life by any definition.

Recovery is Possible for All

If this body wasn't mine, would I still hate it?
~ Danny-J

It is my belief that recovery is possible for all.

It is also my belief that recovery is not only possible but inevitable, once you have what you need.

No one's natural state is an ED. No one willingly chooses an ED when they are capable of a better choice. No healthy, happy, fulfilled, and fully functioning human being chooses to starve themselves to death.

A dysfunctional relationship with food is only ever a reflection of a dysfunctional relationship with yourself.

You can live without the ED but only when you learn how.

Recovery is Your Choice

> *By not making a decision, you are making a decision.*
> *~ Silke Herwald*

I know, as great as it is to imagine not being consumed by this illness, I also know choosing recovery is still scary beyond belief. I know recovery doesn't always feel like the right choice, but now is your time to consider getting real about recovery, because until you do, this illness is not going anywhere.

Recovery does not happen through magic, hope, by accident, or in the background of a busy life.

If you want anything for yourself outside of the suffocating confines of life with AN, you must take a risk in choosing recovery long before you know that it is all going to work out.

If you decide to experiment with changing your life, you can change your life.

This is recovery.

An experiment.

Recovery is Only Ever Meant to be Temporary

> *When you find yourself in hell, keep going.*
> *~ Winston Churchill*

Have there been times or are there still times when you feel the fight will never end? I know I certainly had moments when what I was fighting for felt bitterly pathetic in comparison to the overwhelm of the moment. There were times when any notion of a "healthy" future was unimaginable or trivial, and in no way could I have comprehended that even if it did exist it could possibly be worth *this*.

I know that when you are consumed by the blood, sweat, and dirt of the daily fight that is life with AN, the fact that there is a better life on the other side feels like a fantasy not worth getting your hopes up over.

In those moments, consider keeping the words of this book always in your mind. Because in recovery, there is no question that you will have to experience pain, but the whole idea is that this is short term pain. Pain with purpose. In recovery, you are trading short term pain for long term wellbeing.

Recovery is a means to an end, not a place to live your life.

It is "That Bad"

Wishing it wasn't so doesn't make it not so.
~ Bonnie Killip

Have you ever found yourself telling yourself that it's not "that bad"?

The reality is, when you are living with an ED, there are mediocre moments, there are good moments, and there are phenomenal moments. Life isn't agony a hundred percent of the time.

Which means you're right; it's not "that bad".

But if you consider that without recovery you will continue to be unable to choose your response and never be fully present, that you will never have access to the totality of who you are and that you will never fulfil your dreams, potential, or ambitions, that, most of all, you will never get to simply be you, then I'd say it is "that bad". I'd say it's worse.

Make the Hard Choice

The unknown is too vast to live in known unhappiness.
~ Russell Eric Dobda

You will never feel a hundred percent ready to recover.

I can assure you that the day you wake with the ED telling you it is now time to recover and steps aside as you do so will not come.

Only you can choose it.

You Are Ready, Now

Right here, right now is where you heal.
~ Bonnie Killip

You deserve recovery, and total recovery is achievable for you.

Your one precious life awaits, and you have the chance now, like never before, to begin to make it magical.

You are worthy.

You are enough.

You are *Ready, Now*.

1.2 Overview of Anorexia Nervosa

In the next few pages, I will give a simplified overview of the science behind what anorexia nervosa is (and is not) and how and why some people develop it while others do not.

What is Anorexia Nervosa?

Anorexia Nervosa is an illness, a biopsychosocial illness. This means there are biological, psychological, and social components which contribute both to its development and its persistence.

AN is classified as a restrictive eating disorder in which an individual is unable to consume adequate foods to meet the physiological and psychological needs of their body.

*Note: AN is not who you are, nor is it something which belongs to you, and it is for this reason that I refer to AN throughout this book as "the" ED rather than "your" ED.

Two Subclasses of AN:

1. Restrictive subtype in which you engage in purely restrictive eating patterns
2. Binge/purge subtype in which you alternate between restrictive eating and consuming large volumes of food (binging) in addition to self-induced vomiting or overuse of laxatives and/or diuretics.

In both subtypes, it is common for a person with AN to compulsively engage in excessive exercise (exercise beyond what is healthy for their body).

Core Psychopathology: Misidentification of Food as a Threat

At the centre of the illness process is the brain's misidentification of food as a threat. To explain what this means, I'll start by describing what normally happens in the brain of healthy people when we eat.

In healthy people, eating activates a pleasure-reward pathway in the brain. The activation of this pathway generates feelings of pleasure and enjoyment. This is a physiological adaptation that has evolved to encourage us to eat by rewarding us for doing so. Evidently, it is an incredibly important adaptation, because without this physiological response, we might not consciously always remember to eat enough, and not eating enough clearly poses a problem, as it is incompatible with life.

Eating to the nutritional and energy needs of your body is a central part of survival, let alone the next step up; health.

In people with AN, the wiring of this pleasure-reward pathway is disrupted. The neural pathways that would usually signal hunger and the drive for finding and eating food in healthy individuals are altered[2] in such a way that the thought or act of eating causes a response of extreme fear and intense anxiety[1] or panic.

It's Not "Just" Food

> *Cowards confine themselves to what they know to be true.*
> *~ Anastasia Broder*

Explaining this pervasive fear of food and eating is difficult because it is beyond the realm of comprehension of a healthy person that something as benign, necessary, and, indeed for healthy people, pleasurable as food could elicit such intense fear.

One way I have heard this rewiring of the brain that results in food being misidentified as a threat described was when a guest dietitian lecturer presented a lecture on EDs during my Nutrition and Dietetics degree. The presenter said when he was attempting to explain to parents the huge fear their child with AN has of eating, he found it useful to ask the parents to imagine their biggest fear. I encourage you to do this exercise now if you would like to gain some insight into what your loved one is going through or would like to be in a position to offer more compassion if you work with people in recovery from EDs.

For example, your biggest fear may be having to swim with sharks, being locked in a room full of spiders, or falling from a great height. Imagine a situation that gives you an adrenaline rush, sweaty palms, and the compulsion to escape and get as far away as possible as quickly as possible. If there is something that causes you to lose all rational thinking as your body and brain drop into your primal freeze, fight or flight instincts—ultimately, the thing which brings up the biggest fear response in you—choose that thing.

This is on par with how terrifying it is for your loved one to face the prospect of eating.

You probably noticed your fear response happen long before you got to decide how you'd like to feel or respond? This is the case in anorexia nervosa also. Your loved one's logical mind eventually comes on board to rationalise it out, make sense of it, and decide there is no real threat (this is harder to do when we are starved or malnourished, which we will delve into in more detail later). However, what I want you to begin to get an appreciation for is the fact that our bodies respond long before we truly, consciously know what's happening or why it's happening.

Fear is not a conscious choice.

With this in mind, you can certainly appreciate how much trust your loved one is placing in your hands when you are asking them to face this fear and sit down to eat food six times a day or more.

It's Not About Weight

Saying you understand anorexia because you've dieted a few times is like saying you know what it's like to be decapitated because you've had a paper cut.
~ Anon.

AN is not being "afraid to gain weight". Consciously, people with AN often want to gain weight and understand the health implications of starvation and malnourishment, but the fear is unconsciously preventing them.

Someone with AN may justify this fear in a desperate attempt to have it make some kind of sense to themselves or others.

We feel the need to come up with logical explanations for the illogical fear of food, and it is fear of weight gain which seems most logical. After all, many otherwise rational people in Western society don't want to put on weight or become "overweight" because our societal messages are strongly opposed to living in a larger body. Diet culture is insidious but that's another book in itself.

However, what you need to appreciate is that these feelings are not the same as what you or your loved one living with AN experience. The feelings and experience of living with AN are incomparable to those of an otherwise healthy person with weight, body image, or food issues, because, while there is no question that all these are life disrupting, draining, pointless, and unarguably unfair, AN is not weight, body image, or food issues—it is an illness. AN is a debilitating, all-consuming, and life-threatening illness.

Why do Some People Develop Anorexia Nervosa?

The development of AN is considered complicated and multifactorial. Current evidence shows a strong genetic component,[3-6] with twin-based heritability estimates of fifty to sixty percent[7-12].

A recent study compared the genomes of almost seventeen thousand people with AN to the genomes of over fifty-five thousand healthy people and found significant genomic differences in eight gene areas (called loci)[13] involved with energy and fat metabolism, other psychiatric problems, and physical activity.

What This Means and Does Not Mean

This does not mean that those born with a genetic predisposition will inevitably go on to develop the illness. What it does mean is that those with the genetic predisposition are at higher risk of developing AN if they are also exposed to triggering environmental factors[14-17].

What Are Triggering Environmental Factors?

Triggering environmental factors are events or circumstances which result in a period of energy deficit (inadequate food being eaten).

Circumstances which may lead to inadequate food intake include but are not limited to dieting or intentional weight loss as is often assumed. Inadequate food intake can occur for any number of reasons, including increased energy needs during growth; increased exercise without a corresponding appropriate increase in food intake to support this; trauma; illness which limits food intake for a time; and in some cases, even things like the removal of wisdom teeth and having to consume only liquids can be a trigger.

Whatever the reason for the inadequate energy intake, this appears to be an essential factor in contributing to triggering the onset of the illness.

Crucially, the bodies of people with a genetic predisposition toward AN respond to a negative energy balance differently than the bodies of those who do not have a genetic predisposition for this illness.

Other Factors Contributing to the Development of Anorexia Nervosa

There is also increasing evidence that there are certain personality characteristics or what we'd consider "traits" that may further contribute to why some people are at higher risk of developing EDs. There are four specific traits identified to be highly correlated with EDs, namely perfectionism, harm avoidance, anxiety, and inhibition[18].

In a person with these traits and a genetic predisposition to AN, the development of AN can be triggered by the person's use of controlling food intake and/or increasing exercise as coping strategies to deal with trauma or even what we may consider "normal" life stresses. These same behaviours may also be initiated not as coping strategies but with well-meaning intentions to become healthier, be good, lose weight, or abide by the rules and health messages of their family, peer group, school, the media, society and so on.

In people who are predisposed to AN, these coping strategies, attempts to be healthier, get things "perfect", or be "good" can become increasingly extreme and progress to the pathological state of AN, in which the neural pathways and therefore the structure and function of the brain are altered.

At this stage, the individual's behaviours are no longer carried out through freewill or because of the original initiating conscious intention (if there was one, because I also want to make clear that a lot of our decisions are made unconsciously, and this is often the case for people who develop anorexia nervosa. I just happens). Now, the behaviours have become unconscious and are completely outside the control of the individual. Meaning, what may have started out as a means of gaining more control in a world that is terrifying and confusing (also incredible and wonderful but undeniably difficult) has moved into a loss of control over something as seemingly simple as food choices.

At this stage, the loss of choice it is an illness.

The Initiating Factor is Not the Illness

I feel it is necessary to briefly reiterate that there is a difference between the illness and the initiating factors or situation that enabled the illness to enter someone's life in the first place. There is a profound distinction between the two, and it is only through understanding this distinction that appropriate treatment can be pursued.

AN can start because of any number of reasons, a few examples of which I gave above, but what is important to be clear on is that the initiating factor is not the illness. AN is not the striving to be thin or beautiful—it is an illness. Which means that no amount of nutritional education, body positivity, love, or reassurances can cure AN.

All these considerations would definitely go a long way toward preventing many people from doing the behaviours that led to them falling sick in the first place, and I'm not discrediting the importance of any of them, but none of them will heal the person once it has progressed to an illness.

What it actually takes to recover is going against what feels right and natural to the person living with AN, and that's a whole different ballgame.

Summary to Overview of Anorexia Nervosa

AN is a brain-based illness in which the neural pathways of the brain are pathologically altered in such a way that food evokes an intense and unconscious (automatic) fear response (freeze, fight, or flight). As a result, the person loses the ability to self-regulate and becomes unable to consume adequate food to meet the energy and nutritional needs of their body.

The onset of the illness, in most cases, appears to be due to a genetic predisposition in combination with a period of insufficient energy intake. Certain personality traits have been identified which may heighten the risk of developing the illness.

After the onset of the illness, the thoughts, feelings, and, consequently, behaviours of the person in response to food and exercise are no longer within the individual's conscious control. This means the person is not consciously choosing to eat less, over exercise, or to lose weight. They consciously want to be doing other behaviours but find themselves unable to do so.

Part Two
Psychological and Physiological Aspects of Anorexia Nervosa

To call anorexia an eating disorder is like calling cancer a cough.
~ Prof. Arthur Crisp

Now that you have a brief understanding of what AN is (a brain-based illness) and how someone develops this illness (much like any other illness—a combination of genetics, personality traits, and environmental triggers), I would like to devote this next section to delving deeper into the psychological (mental) and physiological (physical) changes that occur within a human being as they are living with AN.

There are many changes and strange experiences your body and mind will go through both in the depths of AN and in recovery from AN which simply do not happen to human beings who have not lived with the disease. This is because the level of stress that starvation and malnutrition place on a human body and psyche is monumental. This section is to prepare you for some of the things you may expect or to assist you in understanding what may already be happening within your body and mind.

2.1 The Psychology of Anorexia Nervosa

What a wonderful thought it is that some of our happiest days haven't even happened yet.
~ Ann Frank

Introduction to the Psychological Aspects of Anorexia Nervosa

Giving the definition of AN as an illness in which someone restricts food intake feels strange to me, and you may have noticed how small a section of this book I devoted to that diagnosis in comparison to the remainder of the book. This is because this explanation provides minimal if any insight into the extreme mental suffering, fear, and disconnect from one's own sense of self, which is required to permit a person to go against their most essential human survival instinct; the need to eat.

AN, as with any ED, is about so much more than a person's relationship with food.

Disordered Eating is But One Symptom

Have you ever been sick with the flu or a cold? Imagine the disordered eating of someone with an ED as analogous to one of the many symptoms you experience when you have the flu. For example, when you are sick with influenza, you have a runny nose, a stuffy head, a sore throat, aching muscles, lethargy, a cough, irritability, and itchy eyes. Amongst other unpleasant symptoms.

The disordered eating of someone who has AN is comparable a runny nose. It is neither their choice to have that runny nose nor is the runny nose the whole illness or indeed all we want to treat or heal.

Illness Process – Inside the Mind

In this section, I am going to attempt to give insight into what it feels like to live with AN, because a Google search, an entire medical degree, and even the most recent copy of the *Diagnostic and Statistical Manual of Mental Disorders* (DSM) cannot give you this.

However, please know that to capture in words the full horror of what it means to live with AN would be impossible. I don't make an attempt to do so for two reasons, one being the fact that you or your loved one's experience is not mine; you are unique. And two, your healing isn't found in understanding what it feels like to live with anorexia nervosa, your healing is in learning what it feels like to live without AN. That's what comes in the later pages, and it is what the majority of this book is dedicated to.

But to start with, I am going to share what you won't find on WebMD about living with AN, because people who have not lived with an eating disorder find it incredibly hard if not impossible to relate, and people living with an ED more frequently than you'd imagine do not identify with having an eating disorder or feel incredibly ashamed and alone in their experience because of their own misunderstanding of what an ED is. I hope if this is you that what I share here will help you feel less alone or broken.

Two Stages of the Illness Process

When I reflect on the years I spent sick, I see two distinct stages; that of the early stages of naivety, which now as a dietitian and clinical hypnotherapist I see described by doctors in their new patient referral letters to me as "denial" or "apathetic"; and that of the later stages, characterised by a full blown desperation, of wanting to change but feeling entirely unable to do so.

In this section, I will first describe what it feels like to be in the grips of AN, to be living completely at the mercy of what it demands, largely before you become aware that it is a problem. Hint: this stage feels like nothing short of being possessed, and therefore I will aptly refer to it as "possessed".

To give you a brief prelude to what I mean by these two stages, consider this scenario: When I developed AN, I had never heard of it. I had never heard of any form of ED. I didn't know people could have such problems. I had no idea what was happening or that anything I was or wasn't doing was a problem. AN quickly became my "normal".

In the second half of this section, we are going to have a look at the experience of being in the depth of the illness. That is when you are acutely aware of all that is wrong. You learn and understand that you are living with a mental illness, and you may fluctuate between believing you are sick and thinking it's not that bad, but either way you have moments of very much wanting to change but feeling unable to. This is an incredibly confusing and cruel position to find yourself in, which I refer to as "insight but inability to change".

Let us begin with the early stages of the illness.

1. The Early Stages – Possessed

Not Denial but Delusion

In the early stages of the illness, it's not denial, it's delusion.

In denial, you have some understanding of what is going on, but because you know on some level you are ill-equipped to deal with it, you don't.

However, in the early stages as AN establishes its grip, you have no idea why people are making a big deal about your skeletal frame, your miniscule food intake, or excessive exercise. You don't see it as a problem.

I honestly wanted nothing more than for my parents and friends to "get off my back and leave me alone" and for everything to "go back to normal".

Both sentiments I now hear reflected back to me from many of the people I work with who are entering treatment for the first time due to the concern of those who care about them.

You may not even feel you've lost weight, because many people with AN have what is termed body dysmorphia, where they do not perceive their body as the outside world does.

There can also be a complete body mind disconnect, in which case they may avoid looking at or thinking about their body altogether.

In my case, I was for the most part the latter.

I avoided all mirrors and rarely touched, looked at, or thought about my body. I existed almost entirely in my mind.

In hindsight, I was also the former, because while I always "knew" I was underweight, I didn't always feel it or *really* see it. I avoided and ignored it.

I am Different

In the early stages of the illness, you don't know that your food intake is inadequate. It might be the first time in your life you've ever thought about or given attention to what you eat. Even if you can understand that what you're eating would be inadequate for the people you care about, you feel the rules that apply to other people regarding a healthy food intake don't apply to you.

You dismiss it.

You are somehow different.

It's not that you know the truth and are deceiving others so that you can continue with the destructive behaviours, it's that at this stage, you are unaware that the behaviours are destructive. In this stage, the behaviours are saving you from the feelings of inadequacy and uncertainty associated with having no firm identity or autonomy that underly them. They are helping you cope with feelings you may not yet even be able to put a name to.

Often, one of the initiating factors of AN and the need to turn to controlling food begins as an unconscious need to gain a sense of control in a world or situation where you feel you have very little. If you consider for a moment that EDs develop at all ages but one of the common ages for EDs to develop in the teenage years or other times of change or transition it starts to make sense, why. The transition for childhood to young adult to adult are times when the person is supposed to be discovering who they are and their place in the world or advancing who they are. A task which can easily be perceived as overwhelming by those who are highly susceptible to outside influence, wanting to please or get things right.

Outside influence can include when parents or other important people in the person's life are restricting them from exploring, failing, or pushing for them to be "good" in well-meaning ways, such as obtaining good grades, being well-behaved, being mentally more mature than they are, caring for younger siblings, or to excel at sport, and so on.

When you consider the pressures on adolescents, some examples of which I've listed above, it makes sense that the highest risk group for developing AN is adolescent, white, middle-class girls. Of course, this does not mean that this illness is confined only to this group, because having now worked with thousands of people in recovery, I know firsthand that people of all ages, genders, and backgrounds are affected by EDs.

However, AN is more prevalent in adolescent, white, middle-class girls, and I think it's worth exploring why a little deeper, because I believe the generalised characteristics of this population offer significant insight into some of the things that need addressing as a society to lessen the development of EDs. Not just in this population group but overall.

Adolescent girls are educated about the difficulties, pain, and injustices of the world into which they are expected to one day (very soon) become a competent adult.

On top of this is the extreme desire to fit societal norms, including how their body "should" look, the teaching that they are supposed to exist largely to please others, as well as sometimes a lack of capable adults to which they can look up to as competent, resourceful, and inspiring role models. These are the messages you get both overtly and covertly, growing up as a female.

Hence, given that one cannot single-handily fix the problems of the world, fit every societal norm, look like the heavily altered photographs on social media, and please everyone all of the time, people with an underdeveloped sense of self are in the perfect position for everything to go wrong—and sometimes it does.

Sometimes, it goes very wrong.

The Answer Must Be Out There

When I started thinking about the food I ate for the first time in my life, and altering what I ate, I clearly remember looking to the outside world for what to do. I was looking for how to get it right.

This thing that had once felt so easy and come so naturally, this thing I'd never before given a second thought to, now felt like a monumental task.

I became overwhelmed. I was floundering.

I looked first to my younger sister as an example of what to eat. At that stage, she must have been about nine years old. I gave it a go, but she was a fussy eater and not eating enough to be a viable model for my thirteen-year-old self.

Next, I looked to my older sister.

At that stage, she would have been about sixteen years old, and I quickly realised she spent too much time away from our parents' home to be a viable role model for what to eat. She wasn't there enough to copy.

After these failed attempts at mimicking what to eat in fear of getting it wrong and in confusion of what I was supposed to eat, I looked to my friends, I looked to my dad, I looked to my mum, and I looked to magazines. Thankfully social media didn't come into my life until many years later.

I remember reading a magazine in the waiting room of a doctor's surgery that said don't eat after seven p.m. I don't even remember if a reason was given as to why not to eat after seven p.m. I only know from that day on, I never again ate after seven p.m.

I can't imagine what it's like now, with access to billions of bits of information, opinions and products in your pocket telling you how to and how not to eat. Telling you how you should and shouldn't be living your life. Telling you who and what you should and shouldn't be.

In the end, I eventually settled on my mum. She'd always had a strong opinion about eating "healthy" that I'd been aware of throughout my life but had never taken any interest in or given any thought to (consciously that is but more on this later).

I can postulate that for my young mind, she would have seemed like the safest option. If mum ate this, it was safe.

Never once did I look to myself.

I abandoned myself.

Which become a fifteen-year abandonment.

I Must

It is insurmountably both heartbreaking and frustrating to watch someone you love harm themselves in such an extreme way whilst seemingly oblivious or apathetic to the damage they are causing.

What you must understand is that the actions that are part of the illness such as inadequate eating and overexercising are a compulsion. That is; they feel like what must be done, and something that is a *must* is not a choice.

There is no list of options from which they can choose in the way healthy people can. There's not even one alternative. Therefore, there is no ability to decide what they want to do, because the decision is, in every circumstance, premade by AN.

Futureless

The starved, malnourished, overwhelmed, traumatised, and stressed brain is not thinking about the future implications of the harmful actions being undertaken in the here and now.

It is thinking about how to survive the next five minutes.

Many people with AN do not have a clear concept of their mid-term let alone long-term future, or they can imagine no future at all.

When your brain is underfed and your nervous system is overwhelmed, the fear in the here and now overrides all else. I learned after recovery that my inability to plan for my future was a brain attempting to protect you by not planning for a life in a future that is unstable and uncertain. Because why would you plan for a future if it was unstable and uncertain? Why would anyone? Any plan you did make would be a waste of time and energy.

Your finite resources are used in the here and now because that is far more important when your body doesn't know if you're going to live another day. Your brain is all about conserving energy.

A Life of Reaction

Living with AN is living in a state of reaction.

For me, living with AN meant my life was dependent upon what was happening out there rather than inside me.

I had minimal regulatory processes, and the majority, if not everything, I did was in reaction to something done to me.

In the illness, my emotions were governed by the outside world. If something upset me, my response was to not eat and/or run, and to be honest, even when I was extraordinarily happy, the desire to not eat and run was still there because food felt of no importance. Perhaps looking back because I then felt I was "too much". Being exhausted was the only way to quiet my mind and be "less".

"Don't eat" was my unconscious answer to just about everything. AN became a form of numbing for me.

I was completely reactive to what happened in my daily life, and there was always something AN could twist to be a reason to not eat. Everything was a "sign" and confirmation that I didn't deserve to eat. I couldn't eat unless everything was perfect.

I would come home from school in the afternoons, and before I'd allow myself to have a snack, I had to unpack my things, do my homework, take a shower, make sure everything was just right. Eating was the lowest priority on my list (despite thinking about it all the time) and by the time I had things in order and had nothing left to do or distract myself with, I was faced with having the snack, and then suddenly I wouldn't want it.

Perfect never existed, and even if it had, even if I knew what the perfect conditions to eat under were, there would still have been a reason to not.

The overwhelming sense of guilt I felt when it came to feeding myself prevented me. Eating was wrong.

It wasn't something I had to remind myself of or try to not do, it was wrong at the cellular level. This I knew with more certainty than anything else.

Run

Any time I was left home alone, I would have to run.

In my most exhausted moments, when I knew everyone was going out, I would sometimes experience these overwhelming feelings of dread because I was going to "have to" do it.

I had a little circuit behind the house that I would run until they came home, or if I had more time and when I moved out or travelled, the runs would become longer.

It wasn't a choice. It was simply what I had to do.

I can honestly say that I wasn't fully aware that this wasn't a normal thing to do. I was following demand after demand from the ED with no reason or logic. I could come up with logic, because that's what the creative prefrontal cortex (PFC) part of the brain of human beings does—creates justifications for why we're doing what we're doing in order to make sense of it to ourselves and others—but knowing what I know now, none of these justifications were accurate. They were just that; manufactured justifications for something which otherwise made no true logical sense.

The demands of AN and what I had to do progressively became larger and larger and more outrageous by the day, until they were unfulfillable, and the shame and inadequacy I felt as I strived to keep up with them kept me exhausted and unable to function.

I was consumed and obsessed.

My world narrowed.

Panic

One of my most vivid memories of the need to run was when one afternoon after school, my younger sister went for a run and my mum went for a walk with her.

I had every medical opinion under the sun stating that I should not be exercising in the condition I was in. My family found it hard to cope, and they coped in the best way they knew how, which at that point in time meant they had more or less snuck away for this afternoon exercise because they must have decided it would have been exhausting (and impossible) to reason me out of coming. They were right.

When I realised what was happening, within 0.001 seconds, my mind had gone into panic.

I lost it.

I can only describe it as full shut down of all reason.

Something else took over entirely.

I bolted after them.

Starvation and Exercise Feel Good

The same phenomenon is seen in both animals and humans in which exercise releases endorphins and other feel-good chemicals. When your brain is malnourished, these feel-good chemicals are in low supply. Which means exercise offers more than temporary relief from acutely unpleasant emotions, it also supplies some pleasure and, in a world where all you can hope for is temporary relief, that pleasure is indescribable.

The starved brain's increased preoccupation with exercise is also hypothesised to be an evolutionary adaptation supporting the drive to keep on the move in order to find food. The reasoning is that back in the day of cavemen and cavewomen if you were starving, there's clearly no food available in that area, and the logical thing to do would be one of two things; stay still to conserve energy or move more to find food.

Apparently, people who are predisposed to AN fall into the latter category. There's even reason to believe that back in the day they would have made great clan leaders because of this ability to continue under such tough conditions such as famine.

Having lived that experience, this one resonates with me most. It really did feel biological.

It wasn't just running and it's not just structured exercise for people living with AN when we talk about "compulsive exercise" we're also talking about constant low-level movement like spending long periods standing, the desire to constantly keep moving and doing things including cleaning.

However, I believe it's likely a combination of reasons rather than singular as to why people with AN frequently (not always) feel a compulsion to exercise, including exercise being a form of further unconscious distraction in the same way that starvation is a distraction from oneself. When you don't have (or don't perceive you have) the tools, the environment, or the support to deal with the illness (or life in general) distraction is a viable tactic. Recovery then is not so much about removing distractions as it is about creating a self and a life you don't need distracting from.

Who Am I?

AN swamped any ability to do self-care long before I even knew the term self-care.

Nothing was about me.

I didn't know what self-care meant because I didn't know what "I" meant.

I would wear the same clothes for days. It's possible weeks. I don't remember. I would go to bed in them, get up in them, go through the motions of a day, and go back to bed in them.

I rarely showered because my body was thin skin just barely covering bones, and the thought of getting naked and cold was unbearable. In any case, I didn't care if I was clean or dirty. I couldn't really feel my body.

I distinctly remember I didn't want to waste the water or soap on myself.

It is inconceivable to me that I once felt this way.

On top of this, everything was a monumental effort.

Every action was painful and exhausting, including getting showered and changed. The smallest of tasks demanded unbelievable concentration, and I often felt I was trying to move through quicksand but in many ways the difficulty was what I found relief in. It quietened my mind and my body.

In a way I believe AN was partly an attempt from my unconscious to self-medicate. Starvation allowed me to dull and quieten an abundance of energy and thoughts I hadn't known what to do with.

Protecting Them

At fifteen I saw my mum breakdown in the dressing room of a clothes shop when I tried on a bikini.

I developed a fear of looking at myself in the mirror.

It wasn't that I couldn't see that I looked thin, I could. It was that I couldn't change it. I also felt disconnected from it like it was someone else's body. I felt I always had to be brave. I felt I had to keep my mum safe from me, to not let her down or disappoint her, because if she was upset and disappointed in me over something so small, imagine how much I'd let her down if she knew the full truth.

During the years I lived with AN and all the years I would have considered myself in recovery, I was doing it for others. Everything I did was with the intention of lessening the pain for others. I never focused on changing the pain for me. It is this which I remember most about all those years. I was more concerned about protecting others than anything else.

With hindsight, it's clear that this was a major factor that likely kept me stuck. My world was reduced to obsessing, worrying about, and trying to anticipate and meet the needs of other people.

I also recognise that when I was sick, I had an inadequate ability to deal with other people's emotions, as their emotions felt the same to me as if they were my emotions. There was no separation. Therefore, I was forever trying to make others comfortable and happy as a means of feeling more comfortable and happier myself. I was trying to control other people's experience of this experience we were all going through.

It didn't work.

Relentless Overwhelm

I was constantly overwhelmed. I regularly felt on the verge of a breakdown. I felt for the longest time that I was *just* holding it together. I was inconceivably fragile but acting so tough because (I believed) no one could help.

I didn't want to be a burden.

I was running off adrenalin.

I was perpetually distracted and exhausted.

There was a constant need to keep moving and a relentless drive to keep doing, which further prevented me from ever looking inside myself to ask the question of what I needed.

I was impossibly hard on myself and had ridiculously tough schedules and rules around everything, including times I could and could not eat, foods I could and could not eat, where and how much and with whom I could eat.

Spontaneity disappeared from my vocabulary.

Unexpected changes to plans or routine triggered monumental panic within me. Panic I had to keep inside because of the immense shame I felt that these things did cause me panic.

Yoga

My mum used to teach yoga classes on the veranda of our family home. When the condition of my physical health made it no longer possible for me to go to school, I would join in and do these yoga classes.

There was always a meditation or relaxation component at the end of the class. During which I would get up and go do schoolwork or lie there and read a book. So complete was my inability to sit even for a minute with my internal thoughts. To do so was to me the greatest waste of time.

I was the greatest waste of time.

Obsession with Food

I was obsessed with food. I was constantly planning and buying food. I would lie in bed in the morning beside my boyfriend agonising over planning each meal for the day just right.

Then, of course, when it came to it, I couldn't eat it.

I would plan and cook meals that were amazing and decadent for others but be too afraid to touch them myself.

At the time, I didn't think this was weird at all.

I never truly hated food; I did fear it though. A lot. The pain of eating it just wasn't worth it.

A Recipe for Disaster: Food and Other People

Every time someone passed up on food or said they didn't like this or that food, I would panic. It tore me apart. I fixated on it, and I could not let it go. Every time someone shared what they'd eaten that day of what they ate in general I would compare. Every time I would find myself adding a new rule to my impossibly large list of rules. Every time I would find myself lacking.

On the other hand, seeing people enjoy food or eat as though it was no big deal gave me a high. The feeling of relief I got when other people ate was intoxicating. My fascination with what other people ate equally so.

The relief was only ever temporary though, because a part of me could never quite believe that other people were fine.

I was hypervigilant and always looking for cracks in the "act", because it was unfathomable to me that people could do this naturally.

Fun?

I read cookbooks for "fun" when I was fourteen years old.

Fuelled by my food obsession (another biological adaptation to starvation), I developed a monumental cooking knowledge and aptitude.

By the time I was sixteen, I'd scoured hundreds if not thousands of recipes and meticulously written out and memorised many.

Recipes I would never eat.

A lack of cooking skills or knowledge was never an issue.

I wasn't looking at the cookbooks to eat the food myself, because although I probably did want to, I didn't know I wanted to, and even if I did know I wanted to, when it came to it, the follow through of putting that stuff in my mouth was impossible.

I had rules in place to prevent me from doing anything that was "bad" or "wrong", and those rules were gospel. They were black and white, and if it was a food or a time when I couldn't eat, I wouldn't even consider it.

It was just the way it was.

Sticky Date Pudding

At about 15 years old I went with my parents to buy a new stove. One of the two stove options they were deciding between came with a free cookbook. I was sold. I spent the rest of the shopping expedition thinking about that book. Thinking about the mesmerising glossy cover photo of sticky date pudding, of the pages filled with other rich and decadent foods I could no longer comprehend eating.

I hoped and hoped they would buy that stove so I could read that book. So, I could make that food and not eat that food.

The World is Full of Places to Hide Food

I would scrape butter off bread and under my fingernails. I would smear yoghurt up the side of my bowl. I would spit food into tissues or down my sleeves, pretending I was wiping my nose. I would hold food in my mouth until I could walk away and spit it out. I was forever finding screwed up balls of unidentifiable mould-riddled food weeks later in my clothes' pockets, bags, and hiding around the corners and crevices of my room. I never decided to do these things.

I had no idea why I was doing these things.

The Disappearing Sandwich

The small period of time in which I made my school lunch became the most confusing task in the universe.

I made a sandwich one morning and realised I could leave the cheese off.

The next morning, I realised I could leave the egg out.

I ate the sandwich with avocado, lettuce, and beetroot.

The next morning, I realised I could leave the beetroot out.

The next morning the avocado.

At school I ate a sandwich that was bread and lettuce.

The next morning, I realised I could simply pack nothing, because a sandwich to me now meant bread and lettuce.

What was the point?

It never occurred to me to add things back in.

Wrong

I knew eating was wrong. With every fibre of my being and every cell in my body, I knew it was fundamentally wrong.

The emotional torment that exploded inside me as I watched someone serve food that I "had" to eat was indescribable.

I felt like punching them, shouting, breaking the plate.

I felt like scratching out my eyeballs.

I felt like peeling off my skin.

I felt like banging my head against the wall.

I felt like running and running and running and never returning.

Health, losing weight, or what my body looked like did not come into it.

Stuck: A Tribute to Anorexia

To be in the depths of AN is the definition of stuck. In this initial stage of the illness, you don't fully know it because you still believe that in some way you have control. You may even still be questioning if you are indeed even sick, and there's a part of you that still thinks that when you really want to change, you can.

When I was a couple of years into the illness, my older sister said that it takes on average four years for someone to recover from AN (I have no idea where this figure came from, and the most recent one I've seen cited is seven years. Wow). At that stage, when she said that, I didn't really identify with having AN (mostly because even after living with it for years, I still didn't really know what it was), and if I did, there was no way it was going to take me *that* long.

Almost fifteen years later, I knew different.

2. In the Depths of the Illness – Insight but Inability to Change

From my experience, both personally and professionally, one of the things which characterises AN and is exceptionally confusing and frustrating both to live it and to be on the outside trying to help is that people with AN often possess incredible insight into the illness and what they "should" be doing, while simultaneously showing a complete inability to do it.

This felt like being at war within myself.

There is a profound psychological torment that comes with wanting to stop doing all the ED stuff so badly but at the same time being incapable of following through with better actions. I wanted to stop, but at the same time there was a part of me which felt completely out of my control, and for a long time this part was the larger and stronger part.

The larger and stronger part didn't want to stop because it truly didn't know how to stop. Most of all, it didn't know another way of being.

When "Natural" is Unhealthy

The thoughts and beliefs that lead to the ED behaviours become so deeply ingrained that your brain structure is altered. They become your natural way of being.

That's how pervasive this illness is.

In moments of peace and reflection, the thought of stopping feels alluring and the thoughts of recovery and health exhilarating. However, in the heat of the moment, to do anything differently feels worse than death. In the heat of the moment, you find yourself reverting automatically to the ED coping behaviour without even realising it, let alone knowing why.

This is truly the time in which the illness feels like a monster. You don't want to be doing any of it anymore. You know better. You want better. You are deeply ashamed of your actions. Yet you are, for all intents and purposes, powerless to change, because what feels right, what comes naturally, is the very thing you are trying to change.

Mind Games

I would take food out of my bowl and hide it. Only to try to sneak it back into my bowl a few minutes later so that I could eat it. Sometimes I would do this repertoire of removal and put back four or five times during a meal. It was the most confusing and humiliating experience. I wanted to eat, but at the same time, I was terrified to eat.

Part of me didn't want to eat it.

Part of me wanted to eat it.

The fight would go back and forth in my head in a never-ending cycle of desperation and confusion, until I was completely and utterly exhausted. Overwhelmed and ashamed by the absurdity of my situation and the threat of the seemingly insurmountable task ahead.

I didn't understand why. I didn't understand *what* was wrong with me. All I understood was that *there was* something deeply wrong with me. I was broken and, in my mind, I was broken beyond repair.

I was living in an almost perpetual state of exhaustion, fear, and confusion, where nothing felt real. Nothing felt safe or trustworthy. I couldn't even understand or trust myself to meet my most basic human need for nourishment. This meant the rest of the world was frightening beyond what I can, now that it's over, fully appreciate.

Toast: Now a Quick Snack Once Upon a Time Both Heaven & Hell

Everywhere you go, there you are.
~ Confucius

The first time my mum really spoke with me about "it", she made me a piece of toast laden with butter and jam.

I remember how pathetically grateful I felt. I thought, *This is the end of the pain*. I thought, *This is my recovery*. I thought, *I won't have to live like this any longer* (whatever "this" was). I thought it was over.

I thought wrong.

The confusing thing was that even as I was bursting with gratitude for that piece of bread, and most of all toward my mum for giving me the permission to eat, I simultaneously wanted to rip it up and smush it into the ground with my foot. I wanted to yell into her face that I hated her.

In no uncertain terms, I wanted to die.

I wanted to scream and run out into the night and run and run and run and never stop.

The only problem with the reaction of running and avoiding (which I did follow through with many days and nights to come) was that at some point, you realise that no matter how fast or how far you run, you can't outrun yourself.

There wasn't a thought process behind it.

There was no desire to not eat the calories or not get fat or anything along those lines. This was many years before I learned what a calorie was. My response had nothing to do with the part of my logical, rational mind that could conceive of calories. It wasn't generated from that place. It was a pure and primal fear response.

It wasn't a choice, because my choice as a human being would have been to eat the entire loaf of bread, as my body was screaming for (as any healthy but otherwise starved human being would), but I had to compose myself and control myself.

AN was always about being "normal", fitting in, being "good", staying within the lines and absolutely not rocking the boat.

My mum had given me one piece of toast, and to me, that meant I was deserving of and needed only one piece of toast. Without question.

We're Just Getting Started (#593 of Things Your ED Doesn't Say)

Years after the toast incident, I moved out of my family home, and there were many, many more conflicting and exhausting moments with food to come.

My relationship with food became such that I would either be force-feeding myself or starving. There was little middle ground.

I have memories of how traumatic this was as a woman in my early twenties, sitting on the floor and crying through every mouthful of some food or other.

I have so many memories of endless self-imposed pep talks in readiness for dinners with my partner's parents, with friends, and with my family. All people I genuinely loved and cherished and wanted to connect with, but there was always the fear.

Everything and anything I did was tainted with fear, and the more I tried to get better, the more desperate, helpless, and ashamed I became when I couldn't.

The thought of having to feed myself every day for the rest of my life petrified me.

My Sister's Wedding

I flew from Panama to Germany for my sister's wedding.

On her hen's night, her mother-in-law made a capsicum cheese soup, which was the richest and most flavoursome thing I had eaten in an impossibly long time, perhaps years.

I was distraught.

I couldn't eat it, but I had to in order to be polite.

Food was so much more than food.

I didn't want to let my sister down.

Eating that soup felt like death by a thousand cuts.

I collapsed on my bed after. I was so cold, confused, hungry, and sad. I wanted to curl into a ball and never move again. I wanted to be happy and joyous for my sister, but I had lost my mind.

A couple weeks later, our mum flew in, and one evening we took a train to explore a gorgeous little village.

We got somewhat lost.

It got dark and past my arbitrarily designated "dinner time".

I was thrown into the midst of internal chaos, of which I don't think is possible to recreate from a mind that is not consumed by AN.

I shut off and walked ahead. Fast. I cried and was utterly unable to communicate with any semblance of a rational human being. With my head down, I marched as if trying to get to some unknown destination or some future time where the pain would stop.

I was twenty-five years old by this stage, and while I may have gained greater maturity and insight into AN, it didn't help. In a way, it made it all worse because it added to the shame.

Now, looking back, I know my starved, sick mind interpreted that situation to mean my mum and sister did not love me or care about me, and if that were true, my response was pretty reasonable; however, it wasn't true.

It was just the story my brain consumed by AN fed me.

Today, I am able to look back on that incident and many others like it with boundless compassion myself. However, at the time, I didn't have that understanding. I certainly didn't offer myself any semblance of compassion. In the moment, I wished I was dead, so all-consuming was the level of loathing I felt towards myself.

Most of the memories I have with my sister in the weeks leading up to her wedding were dominated by the fear she wasn't eating enough. That was what I cared about most.

IQ ≠ Emotional Intelligence

I was an intelligent person. I was an incredibly high achiever, and I thought perfectionism was something to strive for in every endeavour.

I was a straight A+ student, and to share that I couldn't feed myself, that even the thought of feeding myself terrified me, was ludicrous.

There was nothing more humiliating then when my boyfriend at the time and I would have a fantastic, logical, reasonable talk, and I would come out of it exhausted but inspired that I could eat, and then the time would come to eat, and I couldn't.

I couldn't do it.

The fear would be all consuming. It was all I could feel. There was no point at which I could have interrupted it, lessened its onslaught, or chosen to feel any other way. Once the emotions took over, I would be distraught and inconsolable. I would find myself on the floor in full body paralysis. For days.

That's the unembellished degree to which this took over my body, mind and soul.

I hardly even felt human anymore.

Every bit of hope and innocence I'd ever had was gone.

Knowledge is Not Power

I understood well the medical implications of starvation, malnutrition, and being severely underweight. I was always striving to gain weight and eventually invested a great deal of time and effort into learning about what AN was from a medical perspective.

I became an expert in human health and nutrition and completed a degree in Biomedical Science and a double degree in Nutrition and Dietetics, both during the time I was sick.

It was a borderline perverse fascination of mine that it didn't matter how much I learnt and understood about how damaged I was and what was happening to my body, I still couldn't change.

I could sometimes change my actions through sheer force, willpower, and determination, or shame or to protect someone else (guilt), but it always felt wrong to eat.

When you are living with AN, eating is so much more than simply eating. When you are living with AN, food, hunger, eating, every action, every word, everything is interpreted in ways that prevent you from eating.

Which prevents you from living.

It feels like one of those quizzes with the yes/no answers and you take a different path according to your answer, but with AN, any and every path you take leads to the "don't eat" box.

Slashing at Shadows

I had many more years in this second stage of AN with the full awareness that my body was suffering and trying to change than I did time in which I was completely under the delusion of AN.

During this time, when I was aware of what was going on, wanting and trying to change, I thought I was in recovery.

In hindsight, I wasn't. I wasn't capable of recovery.

I knew I had an illness. I knew I wanted to get better. I was trying everything I was told would help me to get better. However, what I didn't know was that this isn't the same as being in recovery.

I was fighting and fighting and fighting, but I was fighting the wrong thing in the wrong place with the wrong tools.

I was slashing at shadows and an enemy that did not exist.

I was fighting myself.

Conclusion to the Psychology of Anorexia Nervosa

Like an abusive partner, AN keeps you in an almost constant state of confusion, exhaustion, and overwhelm. You are so scattered and disconnected from your true self and from the rest of the world that it's hard to know which way is up or down.

You question everything.

You're much easier to control from there.

Which is why I want you to know that in the same way that you get a sore throat when you have a cold and it heals when you get better, these thoughts and behaviours that are symptoms of the illness that is AN will leave with your recovery.

Until, one day, quite by surprise, when you're no longer fighting for it or even looking for it, you realise you simply no longer feel any of those old ways you once felt.

You simply no longer do any of those old things you used to do.

Now that we've discussed illness process from a psychological perspective, let us look at some of the ways in which an inability to eat affects your physiological functioning and further amplifies and perpetuates the psychopathology of AN in a vicious feedback loop.

2.2 The Physiology of Anorexia Nervosa

There is a vast array of medical complications associated with AN, all of which are related to weight loss, starvation, and malnutrition[19].

Introduction to the Physiology of Anorexia Nervosa

I recognise that knowing the medical implications of starvation and malnutrition alone will not change your capabilities and lead to recovery.

As I've shared within the previous chapter, I've been there. I know what it feels like to know all the things that are wrong with you and to try to use them as "motivation" to get better, to do better, to be better and have it change nothing.

Therefore, if you would prefer to skip this section (if it's going to be demotivating or overwhelming rather than useful for you) and go straight to Part Three and the recovery section, please feel welcome to do so.

You don't need to know everything that's wrong in order to get better.

Much of what is happening for you now, you will only fully appreciate on the other side of recovery. Which is why the information in this section is designed to be especially useful for those caring for loved ones as well as health professionals working with those in recovery, perhaps more so than it is useful for those living it.

Note to Carers

Your loved one is stuck.

Logical medical information can and certainly is used in the hope that it will scare people into eating better and this may work temporarily, but it is only ever going to be temporary. Forcing yourself to eat out of fear is not the same as being able to naturally eat well. Fear is not a lifetime strategy for eating, because fear is not a strategy for a lifetime of health, happiness, or fulfillment.

It is my intention that if you, as a carer for a loved one or as a health professional, have a good understanding of how serious the physiological implications of this illness are and how necessary it is to seek good treatment for your loved one, beyond getting them to "just eat", and how much they need your help to access treatment, you will be proactive in ensuring that your loved one gets the best help now.

There is no greater way you can help than to get them the treatment they need, because medical stabilisation and all the support, love, compassion, empathy, or attempts at lessening their psychological distress will not heal them.

Until they face the underlying issues, the illness isn't going anywhere. Which means one of two things; they either never fully recover, or they die because of the illness.

It really is that straightforward.

Starvation and Malnutrition

Malnutrition

Your biology is based on nutrients, and all these nutrients are ultimately derived from or dependent upon the foods you eat.

Your body has a requirement for a certain amount of three macronutrients (carbohydrates, fats, and protein), thirteen vitamins (for example, vitamin C, B6, and E), and sixteen minerals (for example, iron, magnesium, and sodium) in order to continue functioning.

On top of this, we know there are plenty more nutrients contained within foods such as phytonutrients and fibre which, while not vital for life, provide additional health benefits.

If your nutritional requirements are not being met through your diet, your body uses what it has stored.

When you are eating well, your body stores each nutrient to differing degrees. Some it's able to store well (for example, vitamin B12) and others not as well (for example, vitamin C). However, no matter how well your body stores each nutrient, these stores are finite. Which means in times where inadequate food is being eaten, inadequate nutrition is coming in to replenish them. Therefore, these stores will eventually run out.

When your stores run out, and there continues to be inadequate nutrients coming in, this leads to deficiencies and malnutrition. Malnutrition being the result of a prolonged time over which your body has received an inadequate intake of energy, protein, fats, carbohydrate, or other nutrients, including vitamins and minerals. Deficiencies and malnutrition are serious and can result in permanent brain damage, physical disability, and death.

Starvation

Starvation results from a period of extreme energy deficit, which means not eating enough energy (kilojoules or calories) to meet your body's needs (kilojoules or calories come from foods containing the three macronutrients).

During starvation, there are characteristic physical and psychological adaptations that the human body experiences. All of these adaptations are intended to conserve energy (kilojoules or calories) and prolong survival. These adaptations include lowered metabolism (hypometabolism), lowered heart rate (bradycardia), lowered body temperature (hypothermia), and lowered blood pressure (hypotension).

These energy-conserving adaptations to starvation are your body's attempt at keeping you alive, with the hope that these measures are enough to sustain you until your food intake increases and your body can then use the new nutrients coming in to heal.

Not one of these energy conserving adaptations are designed to allow for a healthy, happy, or thriving life. You can't live a full life under the stress of starvation.

You can barely live.

A Last, Desperate Resort

Your body's first goal during the harsh conditions of starvation is to minimise harm. Next, if insufficient energy continues to come in harm is unavoidable and your body's goal is to simply keep you alive at all costs.

What this means is that, eventually, your body must resort to breaking down your tissues in order to provide the energy and resources it needs to maintain the processes necessary to keep you alive (vital processes).

In this case, the healthiest state your body can keep you in is alive, but it can't do this indefinitely, because your internal organs, including your brain, liver, kidneys, and intestines, as well as your muscles, including your heart, [20] are slowly being broken down.

If inadequate outside sources of nutrition continue to be provided, your body has no other option but to continue this organ and tissue breakdown. The results of which is inevitable long-term and irreversible structural and functional damage and eventually death.

Metabolic Changes

Starvation causes your metabolism to slow down (hypometabolism), an adaptive response to conserve what energy your body is receiving. In order to do this, your non-vital processes are slowed or shut down to conserve fuel for your body's vital functions.

For example, fuel will be conserved for your heart, lungs, and other vital organs versus being used in processes that are not necessary for immediate survival, such as the growth of your hair, reproductive functions, including menstruation, and impaired wound repair.

Fat & Muscle Wastage

Most descriptions of AN include severe weight loss or "underweight" as a defining feature of the illness. However, this is not always a reliable criterion, because the definition of what a harmful level of weight loss is will differ from person to person.

It is well recognised that people with AN can be starved or malnourished at what would be considered a normal or even overweight Body Mass Index (BMI). Furthermore, weight loss does not have to be "severe" for your body to be compromised and to be harmed by starvation and malnutrition.

People with AN do not always look exceptionally thin, or you yourself may be thinking you are not thin enough to be physically at risk.

You are.

If you are not supplying your body with adequate nutrition, you are at risk of all the harms of malnutrition and starvation, irrespective of what the number on the scale reads.

Therefore, I will describe weight loss not in terms of a number or of being exceptionally emaciated but in terms of fat and muscle wastage. Fat and muscle wastage occur when your body is not getting its energy needs met and resorts to breaking down your body's muscle tissue to provide the energy you need to survive.

Normal Metabolism

To explain exactly why it is your body breaks down your fat and muscle—and why this matters—I'll first give a quick rundown of what happens under normal eating conditions:

When you eat foods containing carbohydrates, your body breaks these foods down in your digestive tract to release glucose (or sugar). This glucose is transported into your blood to travel throughout your body and supply energy to your organs, muscles, brain, and every cell of your body, because in a similar way that your car runs on petrol or diesel, glucose is the fuel a human body runs off.

Some of the glucose will be stored within your muscles and liver, where it is linked together into chains of glycogen. These stores of glycogen allow us the luxury of not having to eat 24/7. These stores are what allow us to not starve in our sleep, because while we sleep, our body uses as much as two thirds of our liver glycogen stores.

Essentially, it is from these stores that glucose is released to supply your body with the energy it needs to carry out all the functions necessary in keeping you alive between meals.

When you are undereating, and your body has depleted your glycogen stores, and when inadequate amounts of glucose to meet your energy needs are coming in, your body will move on to using more fat as a fuel. Fat is your body's main storage form for energy. Fat is also more than a source of energy, because it plays a vital role in many other body systems and functions; inclusive of but not limited to your temperature regulation, hormone production, brain function, and protecting your internal organs. What this means is that when you are using your fat stores to depletion, all these systems and the important roles they play are being compromised.

When both your glycogen and fat sores have been depleted and inadequate food continues to come in, your body's last option is to break down protein.

Protein is left until last because, unlike glycogen and fat, it is not stored for use as energy. What this means is that all the protein within your body is serving a purpose. Any diversion of it elsewhere will compromise the functional capacity of your body and cause harm.

Despite the damage being caused as your body increasingly uses your protein for fuel, your body by this stage has no other choice. Its goal is keeping you alive, with the hope that you eat adequality soon and it can then repair the damage it has caused through resorting to using your bodily protein as an energy source.

First, your body will look to pull protein from non-vital sources. Visually obvious signs that your body is resorting to breaking down your protein stores include muscle wastage (noticeable in upper arm and leg muscle loss and sunken cheeks), hair loss, and oedema (for example, puffy ankles).

What is most important to remember is that each of these externally visual signs are indicative of cooccurring internal damage. Including the breakdown of muscle in your digestive tract, making digestion and absorption of nutrients difficult and further compounding the problem of malnutrition.

If your body still isn't receiving adequate protein from dietary sources and the breakdown of these nonvital sources continue, there comes a point where your body must resort to obtaining protein through the breakdown of your vital organs.

This includes the muscle of your heart.

This leads to the integrity and function of your heart muscle becoming increasingly compromised and arrhythmia (irregular heartbeat) are common on electrocardiogram (ECGs) investigation of people living with AN as well as problems with the heart valves, reduced volume of the chambers, and decreased heart muscle mass[21-24].

To put this into context, AN has the highest mortality rate of any psychiatric illness,[25] with a large proportion of these deaths due to heart problems,[26] including weakening of the heart muscle and imbalances in electrolytes.

Electrolyte Imbalances

Electrolytes are minerals, including, potassium, sodium, chloride, and calcium, that are dissolved in your bloodstream and other fluids within your body.

They are responsible in part for regulating and coordinating many crucial bodily processes, including nerve and muscle function, hydration, balancing blood pressure, and repairing damaged tissues.

When electrolyte balance is compromised in people with EDs, due to inadequate intake of foods which are sources of electrolytes, energy production is compromised.

Potassium is one of the main electrolytes involved in the pathway of getting energy into your cells and another electrolyte phosphate in the generation of adenosine triphosphate (ATP), the energy currency of your body.

Depleted phosphate (hypophosphatemia), low calcium (hypocalcaemia), and low potassium (hypokalaemia) in the blood result from prolonged starvation and can all lead to impaired muscle contractility and subsequently weakness, muscle pain, (myalgia) and muscle spasms (tetany).

Low blood potassium, calcium, and magnesium can also impact your heart function. There is something called a Q-T interval, which is essentially the time between when your heart can beat again. This is because your heart beats off an electrical signal and needs time between to repolarise or get ready to beat again. This shows up on an ECG reading as a prolonged Q-T interval.

When the time between when your heart can beat again is lengthened, it means that as your heart rate increases (as it does naturally during exercise or with other heart problems common in those with EDs, including arrhythmias, such as polymorphic tachycardia) your heart may be unable to repolarise before the next electrical signal. If this occurs, it essentially can cause a "short circuit" and sudden cardiac arrest. Which, without immediate medical intervention (CPR, defibrillator, and possibly later drugs and a pacemaker) will result in death.

Bones & Teeth

Stress fractures and broken bones are common in people with AN. Especially in those who engage in excessive exercise, because starvation is enormously detrimental to your bone health.

Young people with AN can often have osteopenia or "thinning of the bones", which may also advance to osteoporosis and bones equivalent to or even frailer than those over eighty years old.

A factor which adds to this problem is that the most common age for people to develop EDs is in adolescence, a crucial time for building bone mass and density.

Peak bone density, that is the strongest your bones will ever be, is generally thought to be reached by the time you are twenty-five years old.

After peak bone mass is reached, natural bone loss of both density and mass is considered a natural part of aging. After twenty-five years of age, the focus therefore is on maintaining or lessening the rate of depletion rather than building bone density any higher. In theory, the higher the peak bone density reached before the age of twenty-five the less the rate of loss as you age will affect the structural integrity and strength of your bones.

The intake of all the nutrients required to ensure the development and maintenance of healthy, strong bones is long and includes adequate protein, calcium, phosphorus, potassium, and vitamin D. All of which are unlikely to be eaten in adequate amounts in people living with AN.

Adding to this is the compounding effects of acidosis (a metabolic result of starvation), which, if it were not for the protective measures your body has in place, would cause your body to become more acidic (incompatible with life).

The protective measures your body goes to in the face of the threat of increasing acidity includes causing the mineral components of your bone (calcium, magnesium, and phosphate) to be broken down to serve as buffers (a chemical which mitigates or pads against the effects of a change in pH). This increased rate of bone breakdown exacerbates and accelerates bone weakening.

Your teeth, in a similar way to your bones, are equally affected by inadequate nourishment. Something which isn't often spoken about in eating disorders is the fact that you do not have to be vomiting in order to damage your teeth. Your teeth are further damaged by acidic breath and changes in saliva composition, which happens when you are eating an inadequate diet, especially a diet low in carbohydrates.

This acidic breath and changes in salvia composition destroys your tooth enamel and causes erosion, cavities, and painful sensitivity.

Hair, Nails, and Skin

Other common manifestations of malnutrition are dull, limp, or brittle hair as well as hair loss.

I had long, thick hair, and it would fall out by what seemed an impossible amount. After each wash, I wondered how I could have any hair remaining. There's something sad and sobering about watching handfuls of your hair fall away every time you shower. My heart goes out to you if you are experiencing this. Don't ignore it and tell yourself it's normal or you deserve it or any other nonsense. It is happening because your hair is made of protein and other nutrients. It takes energy to grow hair, and your body has no protein or energy to spare for non-vital functions.

Protein also makes up your nails and skin. Inadequate protein, energy, and fat intake, together with suboptimal vitamin and mineral intake (such as iron, zinc, and the B vitamins), may cause brittle nails, acne, dandruff, and pale, thin, red, or dry skin.

You may develop pressure sores, bruises, and calluses, especially on your tail bone because of the lack of fat insulating and protecting this area that is under continuous pressure.

You might also find your hands and feet are constantly purplish-blue or feel cold regularly and at times when others aren't as affected by the cold. This is because your body is unable to regulate your temperature properly, leaving your extremities cold, as the blood which would usually circulate through them and keep them warm is being diverted to your vital organs.

On top of this lack of adequate energy, there are a number of mineral deficiencies which can lead to an inability to adjust body temperature in cold environments, including iodine deficiency.

It is common for people with AN to grow longer, fuzzy hairs over their body (most noticeable on your arms and face). This longer hair is called lanugo and is an adaptation by your body to keep you warm because your subcutaneous fat stores have been depleted, which also means your internal fat stores are becoming depleted, which means your body is experiencing huge problems, including disruptions in hormones.

Please note that if your skin has a yellow or orange hue, this can be an indicator of liver damage and requires immediate medical attention.

Hormones and Menstruation

Hormones and neurotransmitters are what keep all the different parts of your body in communication. They are what keep you functioning as a unified whole.

For example, your neurotransmitters allow you to recognise that you have a pain in your toe when you stand on a prickle or to move your hand away from a hot plate, and your hormones allow you to respond appropriately to stress. All these things are outside of your conscious awareness and therefore largely out of your control. They happen immediately in response to external and internal stimuli.

Essentially, these automatic responses have served us exceptionally well in keeping us alive as a species through our evolutionary history. If we had to do this all consciously, we'd be completely overwhelmed before we even managed to get out of bed in the morning.

Our conscious mind is much slower and much more easily overwhelmed than our unconscious mind. Yet, for the most part, as a society we focus on the conscious mind. We predominantly treat people with EDs from a conscious mind framework (more on this later).

Every cell in your body contains fat, and all the hormones your body makes require both fat and cholesterol as crucial structural and functional components. This alone is enough to tell you that having fat in your diet is vital.

In women, loss of menstruation, termed amenorrhoea, or an irregular menstrual cycle is the most noticeable sign that your body isn't receiving the nutrition it needs to create healthy amounts of the main hormone responsible for regulating menstruation; oestrogen.

Menstruation is not a vital part of life at the individual level, and it makes sense that when you're not healthy your body is not going to prioritize growing a baby. In fact, it is no longer an option for your body when it is struggling to keep you alone alive. Therefore, your body will conserve the energy that would go into menstruation or growing a baby by stopping this monthly cycle.

If malnutrition is not reversed in time, it is possible you can go straight to menopause regardless of what age you are. Some women with EDs experience menopause at age twenty. Preventing them from ever being able to become pregnant even if they are to later go on to fully recover from the ED.

Loss of menstruation is important beyond reproduction. It is also a sign that damage is occurring to other areas of your body, including your bones, because estrogen plays a key role in maintaining and promoting bone strength.

If your body is not receiving the dietary fat it needs in order to produce oestrogen in healthy amounts, it means the strength of your bones is being greatly affected, and the same is true in men who are malnourished and not producing adequate amounts of the sex hormone testosterone.

Leptin and Ghrelin

Another adaptation of your body in response to starvation is to decrease production of a hormone called leptin.

Leptin is responsible for signalling to your brain that you are satiated. It is responsible, in part, for creating the feeling that you don't need to eat any more food at that time. The feeling of satiation is different to the feeling of being physically full. Satiated is a feeling of satisfaction or being content with what you have eaten and is influenced by the composition of the food or meal and not just the volume or size of the meal.

Foods or mixed meals higher in carbohydrates, protein, or fat are more satiating than say foods with a high-water content, even though those foods with a higher water content might be larger in size and therefore more filling in terms of physical fullness.

For example, eating seven apples might make you feel physically full but perhaps not satisfied. Whereas eating a sandwich with cheese, mayonnaise, lettuce, and egg might take up less room in your stomach but create a feeling of satisfaction. This is because in the case of the sandwich, your body's needs for the macronutrients (carbohydrates, fat, and protein) have been met.

In comparison, the fruit is low in both fat and protein, and your body is waiting for these in order to send the signal to your brain that your nutritional needs have been met.

The suppression of the hormone leptin is part of what makes you able to eat far more during starvation than if you were well fed and healthy. In starvation, leptin production is suppressed because your body is clever and knows that it needs more food to make up for the period of undernutrition. Your body knows it has a lot of damage to repair, and the faster it can get the materials (nutrients and energy from food) to do this the quicker it can accomplish the task and the lower the risk of long-term damage.

The more you eat the faster your body can heal.

The production of another hormone called ghrelin, which is responsible for hunger signals, is greatly elevated in people with AN (and decreases with weight gain)[27]. This is pretty strong evidence that people with AN are not using willpower to abstain from eating adequately, because it would take levels of willpower no human is capable of to work against all the physiological adaptations your body has to get you to eat (including higher levels of hunger hormones and lower levels of satiety hormones).

Furthermore, of all people, those with AN are the least likely to be capable of generating such monumental willpower, as both components that make up willpower, specifically blood glucose levels (BGLs, or the amount of sugar you have in your blood, i.e., how well-fed you are) and the amount of sleep you've had (or how rested and relaxed you are), are both lacking in people with AN.

The suppression of leptin (decreasing satiation) and the increased production of ghrelin (increasing hunger) are just a couple of examples of the many ways in which your body is desperately attempting to bring and keep your attention focused on food. This food fixation, however, has the opposite psychological effect in people living with AN than what is intended. Instead of the desired outcome of eating more, it causes severe psychological distress and more distrust in your own body, that you are out of control and fear that if you eat you will never stop.

When your body is in starvation, your production of "happy" hormones, including serotonin, oxytocin, and dopamine go down and stress hormones, including cortisol, go up,[28] further adding to your feelings of anxiety and severely impairing focus and emotional stability.

I have worked with many clients who say they never experienced any problems with depression or anxiety until they developed an ED. I also work with many who identify these issues were preexisting but that they were better able to manage them before the ED.

Emotions and Mood

The psychological changes of starvation are due in part to the physical disturbances in hormone regulation and brain function.

People in starvation become angry and impatient, they have a low attention span, display impeded problem solving and a slowed response rate.

When you are hungry are you as kind and patient as you are when you are well-fed? It's likely you answered no to this question (even if it was sheepishly), because the truth is most of us become a great deal more impatient when we haven't eaten well. We have a shorter fuse. Things that may usually not upset us or which we can competently deal with when we are in a fed and calm state are more likely to take a greater time to process and feel more emotional.

This is normal.

This is the way our brains are wired.

When a person is in starvation, this is amplified to the ninth degree, and apathy, low mood, anxiety, and depression are all common in people with AN.

These mood and energy problems, including depression and anxiety, can be due to low protein or energy intake as well as deficiencies in essential fats, vitamins, and minerals. Which means treating these symptoms with antidepressants such as SSRI inhibitors and other drugs is unlikely to offer much in the way of help because if you are, for example, low in the amino acid tryptophan (from protein), you're not going to produce enough of the "happiness" hormone serotonin.

In real life, it is less straightforward than this direct tryptophan to serotonin link, because serotonin production requires more than simply having enough tryptophan in your system. The production of serotonin also requires adequate levels of iron, calcium, vitamin C, folate, zinc, B6, and B3, and if you don't have enough of any one of these vitamins and minerals, you can't make adequate serotonin.

This is the same with the production of each of the hormones and neurotransmitters in your body, they all require their unique collection of vitamins and minerals for proper production and function.

Even if antidepressants did alleviate some of the symptoms, this is not a cure.

Alleviating symptoms is useful as a steppingstone to allowing someone the relief to do what needs to be done, but it is not intended as a long-term strategy.

There is only one thing that will have the desired effect in restoring healthy brain function to someone in starvation and that is nutritional restoration.

You need good nutrition to produce hormones and neurotransmitters in adequate amounts. Therefore, when you are undereating, your body cannot produce in healthy amounts all the hormones and neurotransmitters needed to function let alone feel good.

This is one of the huge challenges of recovery. When we don't feel good or when we are anxious or depressed, eating is often far more difficult and far more stressful than if we felt happy and at ease.

Studies have shown that in individuals with AN, administration of oxytocin is effective in decreasing feelings of distress due to the hypervigilant focus on eating, body shape, and weight[46]. Therefore, it is likely that the poor regulation of mood in those with AN can in part be improved by supporting hormone and neurotransmitter production, including oxytocin, which comes naturally through eating.

At the end of the day, and whatever the underlying processes, your mood and cognitive capacity go hand in hand with your nutritional status.

Starved people are fearful and sad people.

Well-fed people are happy, flexible, and kind people.

Brain Changes

The psychopathology of an ED profoundly affects all levels of your cognitive functioning[29-36].

In those with EDs, brain differences at the level of physical structure in areas responsible for self-regulation, reward processing, and emotional recognition (identifying and understanding your emotions)[37-40] are expected.

In starvation, your body is in a continuous state of stress. In this constant state of stress, you will find it difficult to concentrate, be less interested, engaged, or present, feel lethargic and tired, and generally feel more irritable and shorter tempered than if your brain was well nourished.

Essentially, this is because your brain is focussed on one thing; "how to get food", and the illness is focused on the opposite; "how to avoid food". It's a draining and bewildering twenty-four hours a day seven days a week battle, and, unsurprisingly, your feelings and behaviours reflect this internal struggle.

Studies have shown changes in the brain structure of patients with AN due to the effects of malnutrition, including reduction in grey matter and cortical thinning[41-44]. These changes have huge impacts on our mood and emotional regulation.

I know from personal experience.

I felt as though I was in a constant state of panic.

I was cripplingly unsure of myself and my place in the world and utterly overwhelmed by anything unexpected or confronting. There was no way that I could have coped with the things I do today.

Obsessive, rigid, and repetitive thinking is common in starvation. Your brain is not equipped with the nourishment to reason, and you have very little resilience or problem-solving capability and tend to be at the mercy of strong emotions, which are further exacerbated by constantly low BGLs and nutritional deficiencies.

The process of making decisions, even simple ones, is excruciating and overwhelming, and you get stuck with the simplest of decisions because you want to make the one that is "right" for everyone.

When you are starving and stuck in the illness, you think every decision is of monumental importance, you overanalyse everything (with a brain that is incapable of the task of analysing), which further serves to keep you paralysed in indecision.

I resigned myself to the fact that I just wasn't a good decision maker. The truth is I wasn't a good decision maker, but there was a reason why, and that was that I was starving (and I hadn't developed a sense of self to make decisions from). My brain was in primal survival mode, and I was asking it to function in 21st century life.

No wonder everything felt like the end of the world.

The good news is that the changes in brain structure caused by starvation can be completely normalised. In people following both short term weight restoration and long-term recovery there are no differences between the brains of those who have recovered from AN and those who have never had the illness[45].

Lethargy, Headaches, Dizziness, and Fainting

Lethargy, headaches, light-headedness, dizziness, and fainting are common for people living with AN and can have a number of causes including low BGLs (hypoglycaemia), low blood pressure (hypotension), iron deficiency (anaemia), vitamin B12 deficiency, and dehydration. At their core all these cause stem directly from related to inadequate food intake.

Sleep Disturbances and Insomnia

In healthy humans, BGLs rise after we eat as the glucose from the food is absorbed into our bloodstream. Our bodies then move the glucose into our cells for use as well as storage, and our BGLs are brought back down and always kept within the range our bodies need in order to function correctly (4.0-7.9mmol/L).

Between meals, glucose is mobilised from the glycogen stores (in your liver) and released into your bloodstream. This prevents your BGLs from dropping outside the optimal range.

This system, when functioning correctly, ensures all your organs and body systems are continuously supplied with the glucose they need to function.

When you next eat, those stores can be topped up to again carry you over to the next meal. However, if you are not eating well enough to replenish your glycogen stores and you have not eaten for a prolonged time, such as overnight, your BGLs can fall below 4.0mmol/L. When this happens, you run the risk of dropping into a coma.

Once again, this whole process isn't as simple as eating glucose, because the optimal functioning of the pathways involved rely on a swathe of other nutrients. For example, low zinc and manganese both make you more susceptible to the hormone insulin. Because insulin is responsible for allowing glucose to cross from your blood into your cells, being more susceptible to the hormone insulin can cause extreme drops in BGLs.

It is common for people with AN to experience sleep disturbances. This can include waking up hungry, most often around two a.m. because this is the time at which your BGLs are exceptionally low; your body having used up all the energy from previous meals is waking you up and telling you to eat to prevent your BGLs dropping any lower while you sleep. The danger being if your BGLs were to continue to drop, you risk entering a coma.

If you go into a coma while you are asleep, you can die.

Therefore, if you are experiencing constant waking in the night, get up and have a snack. Preferably fruit or fruit juice immediately, as this is something which is going to get your BGLs back up quickly. Then follow this with something that contains carbohydrate, protein, and fats that will be more slowly digested and maintain your BGLs until breakfast. For example, this could be a piece of bread with cheese, eggs, or peanut butter.

I know the thought of having to eat at two a.m. can be terrifying, but the alternative could very well be not waking up in the morning.

You have so much more to experience in this world to let that be how your story ends.

Furthermore, when you are in starvation or malnourished, your body is prioritising finding food over all else, and this includes sleep. Your body is in a constant state of hypervigilant hyperarousal (stressed), and it therefore can be hard for you to fall asleep or stay asleep, no matter how exhausted you are.

It is also very uncomfortable to lie down let alone sleep when your bones dig into you no matter which way you turn. You have aches and pains everywhere, and your brain offers no moment of reprieve.

Water Retention

Water retention, otherwise known as oedema, is common in recovery.

Oedema causes a puffy appearance of the affected area because water comes out of your blood and into the interstitial cavities.

In recovery, some of the most common places you may experience oedema are around your ankles, legs, and under your eyes.

Oedema has several causes, including low protein in the blood (hypoproteinemia), electrolyte imbalances, hormonal changes, rapid refeeding after prolonged starvation, or low food intake and abuse of laxative, diuretics, and/or diet pills,[47] as well as circulation issues.

Which means the way to rectify oedema is dependent on addressing the underlying cause or causes, which, when it comes down to it, is starvation and malnutrition.

The cure is a regular intake of adequate and nutritious foods, and the key is consistency.

Digestive Problems

The integrity and functional capacity of the digestive system suffers greatly in those with AN, and this manifests in myriad gastrointestinal (GI) symptoms and complications.

Underuse of your GI tract leads to atrophy (wastage) of the smooth muscles. This atrophy means food is emptied more slowly from your stomach into your intestines. The contractions (peristalsis) which propel food through your intestines as well as the production of some enzymes and hormones involved in digestion decrease.

An example of what this means in practical terms is that a meal that would take around 1.5 hrs for a healthy person to digest can take five hrs or more in a person with AN to digest, and bloating, gas, distension, early fullness, nausea, reflux, diarrhoea, constipation, vomiting, and discomfort are common even when eating small amounts of food[48-51]. These uncomfortable and painful symptoms are further compounded by the gut-brain axis, which is acutely sensitive in people with AN.

This stress further reduces digestive capacity, gastrointestinal tract motility, and absorption of nutrients, as the physical processes of digestion are ceased or decreased under stress. This is because your digestive processes are under the control of your parasympathetic nervous system, which takes the lead only when you are in relaxed and calm states, a rare occurrence in recovery, especially and brutally when faced with the prospect of eating.

Cholesterol Disturbances

High cholesterol (total, LDL, or HDL, or all three) is a common finding on analysis of the blood work of patients with AN.

The reasons why are not entirely understood; however, it is thought to be related to low levels of thyroid hormones, a response to malnutrition and starvation in which the cells of your body are being broken down as your body tries to get the cholesterol (your cell walls contain cholesterol and this is then released into your blood and comes up in your test results as "high cholesterol"), protein, and other nutrients it needs to stay alive.

On top of this, there is also evidence that psychological stress increases cholesterol production in your liver[52].

What is most important to know is that in people with AN, these cholesterol abnormalities cannot be corrected through exercise or a low-fat diet (as, unfortunately, is commonly the recommendation by health care professionals who are not knowledgeable in ED treatment). The only strategy that will correct high blood cholesterol is long term renourishment and recovery[53-55].

Conclusion to the Physiological Aspects of Anorexia Nervosa

Change may not always bring growth, but there is no growth without change.
~ Roy T. Bennett

Having lived with AN, you will be depleted in many nutrients, and because it is the interaction of all nutrients which is what is truly important to health, if you were to focus on one specific micronutrient deficiency at the expense of others, you would miss the big picture. Your body needs all the nutrients to function, let alone function optimally.

If you are below the weight your body wants to be (regardless of what you weigh or what your BMI is), and if you're not eating what you need, then your body is suffering.

If you are experiencing any of the symptoms I've covered in this section on the physiology of AN (or any number of others that I didn't include, because this chapter could have easily morphed into an encyclopaedic collection if I were to attempt to do so) it is unlikely that those symptoms will clear up until you are nutritionally restored.

What this means is that you can continue to pursue test after test to confirm your low thyroid function, constipation, food sensitivities, microbiome abnormalities, bloating, intolerances, FODMAP sensitivities, and so on, but until you rectify your nutritional issues and are recovered from the ED, all this is just a convoluted means of distracting yourself from what is really at the core of these issues.

To treat any of these comorbidities as standalone issues will lead you in circles, simply for the fact that they are not stand alone. All these issues originate from nutritional deficiencies, and nutritional deficiencies can only be fixed through full and complete nutritional replenishment.

What many people in recovery don't realise (and I certainly didn't) is that full and complete nutritional replenishment can take years of adequate and consistent eating to fully reverse the damage and for your body to completely heal.

Don't waste time getting caught up in the distractions, because you can spend your whole life there, trying to treat yourself symptom by symptom.

In a state of perpetual malnutrition, you may be eating enough food to maintain weight, enough food to survive, but until you are eating enough food to repair, you're going to continue to have problems.

Get real with the real issue. Get real with the big picture, because when you do, these other problems will often rectify themselves. At the very least, give your body a chance.

What I have covered within this section is by no means an exhaustive list of the symptoms you may experience due to the stress that starvation and malnutrition place on your body. It is, however, my intention to have shone a light on a few things that may be going on internally, with the desire of making it a little less scary and especially to let you know that the damage is reversible and your body will heal.

The one caveat is that your body will heal only when you are able to give it the means to do so (adequate and consistent nourishment along with rest for a consistent period of time beyond what you think "necessary"), and not before.

Now that we have covered some of the psychological and physiological aspects of living with AN, let us now look at the process of providing your body and mind with the means to first heal and then create a new way of living the rest of your life, otherwise known as recovery.

Part Three
Recovery

Nothing ever goes away
until it has taught us what we need to know.
~ Pema Chodron

3.1 An Introduction to Recovery

From the very first page, the focus of this book has been on one goal. That goal is not running from, avoiding, struggling with, battling against, managing, or staying in recovery from AN forever, that goal is a period of recovery and then—recovered.

Recovered is the goal.

This goal can be lost when you are consumed in the day-to-day reality of the battlefield that recovery can so easily become, which is why I want to bring your attention back to the purpose of all this effort and pain, and that is your life on the other side.

You can have recovered. You can be the person you know you can be. The person you truly are. This is available to you. But you can only have it if you are first willing to do the things to get there.

Recovery will be tough, but to reach recovered, you can't skip it. There is no fix without fixing. There is no recovered without recovery.

The Eating Disorder is the Least Interesting Thing About You

It is never too late to choose recovery, and it is also never too early. You are never too sick to recover, and you also do not need to get sicker before you recover.
~ Bonnie Killip

I might not know you personally, but I do know without question that you are unique. I know that there is no one quite like you on this planet.

I also know the ED contributes nothing to your uniqueness or your specialness. The ED is, always has been, and always will be the least interesting thing about you.

I Want More for You

On a personal note, I want you to know that I want more for you. I want you to know that even if you don't yet believe in yourself, I believe in you. I fully, wholeheartedly, and unconditionally believe in your strength to recover.

I believe in you as a unique, beautiful, and competent human being. I believe in that part of you which is pure magic, because even if we often ignore or downplay this part of ourselves in day-to-day life, it undeniably exists. It exists within all of us.

You know it.

We all know it.

I believe not only do you deserve a better life but also that you are capable of living a better life regardless of what you are going through now, have gone through in the past, or are yet to experience.

Recovery Disclaimer

Recovery is taking the hard steps when they are hard, not waiting until they become easier.
~ Bonnie Killip

Full disclaimer: Recovery is more difficult than living with an ED. It can be easy to get caught up in the relief and the promise as you or your loved one chooses recovery, and I believe this is because there is a misguided notion that admitting you have a problem is the hardest part and that when someone does so, half the battle is over.

If recovery were as easy as realising you had a problem, wanting to change and having help to change, people would recover quickly from AN and certainly wouldn't die from this illness.

I have no doubt there are more people sick and wanting to change than there are people who are sick and not wanting to change, because the reality is anorexia is not something you can simply choose to get better from.

Recovery requires an individualised plan, it requires taking purposeful steps, and it requires the courage and faith to continue to follow that plan when it feels like you can't do any of it.

All of which, I assure you, are infinitely harder than the beginning step of merely recognising you have a problem.

Cheers to The Bubble Popper

There are no failures, only feedback.
~ Milton Erikson

Why did I start the section on recovery by sharing that recovery is harder than living with an ED? Because I want you to go into it prepared. I want you to go in with your eyes open, as equipped as you can be, supported and realistic.

Because I went in all gun's blazing, filled with determination and fire that this time I would win. I went in believing that this time I wanted it.

That this time was different.

That this $2,389^{th}$ time was the last time…

Only to be shot down.

Again, and again, and again.

I want you to start collecting the evidence that you are capable of winning, and this means being armed with the reality that recovery includes "failures".

Failures are part of it.

Your failures from your past as well as those you're yet to experience are not proof you are incapable of recovery. Your failures are proof that you are learning, growing, and changing.

Maybe you need to fail four times or two hundred and twenty times to learn that you in fact cannot skip that snack (or whatever other lesson it is).

When you learn from what didn't work and use this information to stop doing those things which are not working and give a new tactic a go, they are not failures at all, they are invaluable and indeed absolutely necessary sources of feedback.

There is No Perfection in Learning

You can do, be and have anything you want in this world as long as you are first willing to become the person who is capable of doing, being and having it.
~ Bonnie Killip

The reality is you won't do recovery perfectly. You can't. Recovery is a messy journey. A messy, heart-wrenching, confusing and overwhelming journey you will only gain an understanding of in hindsight.

Recovery is learning, and there is no perfection in learning.

Recovery is Active, Not Passive

The plan is to change, not plan to change.
~ Bonnie Killip

Recovery is active, not passive. This is because life outside of an ED is active, not passive, and recovery is setting yourself up to live that life. Recovery is setting up the life you want to live, the life you are capable of living, and the life you deserve to live, and action is the secret ingredient that will bring the living of it into existence.

Each miniscule success in recovery matters. Even when you are the only one who can know just how hard it was. Especially when you are the only one who knows how hard it was.

Those little wins that no one else will ever see or ever understand—they are the wins which truly matter.

Your recovery is for you.

On Doing Anorexia

The most meaningful thing you can ever do for your recovery is to close your eyes and think about what it is you want.
~ Bonnie Killip

Before I learned that anorexia was something I was doing (and doing very well), I had always believed I was at the mercy of my emotions.

When I first started practicing having a say over my thoughts, feelings, and emotions and realised it was possible I was excited at the possibilities but simultaneously felt resentment, anger, and deep regret over the years, I had "lost" to AN.

There can be so much regret in the realisation that those years of suffering were needless. Your initial response may be that you want to ignore it or write it off as impossible, positive thinking, too airy-fairy, "but I have an illness, and this is how it makes me think", I have this or that condition that "prevents" me from doing this. "If only this other person didn't treat me this way, then I wouldn't feel or behave this way", or "she doesn't know what she is talking about", and all those thoughts are real and legitimate concerns.

All your fears are valid.

What I want to encourage you to do is consider allowing yourself to begin to entertain the possibility that while all those thoughts are legitimate concerns, they are only serving to give the illness an ongoing presence in your life.

Pause.

Breathe.

And read that again if you need.

By clinging to those thoughts and fears, by justifying and defending them, you are strengthening the bond between you and the very thing you don't want.

To know that over half my life (at that time) had been needlessly consumed by an illness was a big blow to take. Yet it was a learning of which there was no unlearning. Once you know something you cannot unknow it.

I realised I could live in regret, denial, anger, or fear, but if I did, I was lowering the quality of my life in the now and in my future, which are the only parts I now had any control over.

What had happened had already happened. There is no way to undo that. That is painful to know. But it was more painful to consider a future where that become a reason to never change.

To highlight what I mean about choosing our thoughts and the impact this has on our lives, I want to quickly share with you a small tale I first heard from a friend when I was around seventeen years old and very sick.

The Tale of Two Wolves

A Cherokee elder was teaching his young grandson about life.
"A fight is going on inside me," he said to the boy. "It is a terrible fight, and it is between two wolves. One is evil—he is anger, envy, sorrow,

regret, greed, arrogance, self-pity, guilt, resentment, inferiority, lies, false pride, superiority, self-doubt, and ego.

The other is good—he is joy, peace, love, hope, serenity, humility, kindness, benevolence, empathy, generosity, truth, compassion, and faith. This same fight is going on inside you—and inside every other person, too."

The boy thought about it for a minute and then asked his grandfather, "Which wolf will win?"

The elder simply replied, "The one you feed."

~ Tsalagi Tale

I could see how much joy it brought my friend to share it with me.

He loved it.

I hated it.

I hated it because I didn't understand it.

Intellectually, I understood the concept, but I didn't feel it because I couldn't apply it to myself. At the time, I didn't believe my thoughts, emotions, or actions were within my control or that I had choices over what I thought or felt. I believed my thoughts, emotions, and actions were entirely dependent on the outside world and that it was in response to this or that person, thing or situation that I was the way I was.

I believed I had little choice.

I lived as though I had no choice.

I can also look back and see I was in massive denial of the existence of anger, envy, sorrow, regret, greed, arrogance, self-pity, guilt, resentment, inferiority, lies, false pride, superiority, self-doubt, and ego within myself (and other "negative" feelings).

I wanted the world to change.

I wanted the world to be safer and kinder in order for me to feel better so that I could feel different and behave different. I wanted everything and everyone else to be okay before I would allow myself to be okay.

That's one hell of a condition to pin your happiness on.

I came across this small story again by chance recently, and reading it with an entirely new mind, I now think it is poignantly beautiful.

As with many things I believed when I was sick, now, with a completely different understanding, it is a source of constant surprise and delight.

Such things as anger, envy, sorrow, regret, greed, arrogance, self-pity, guilt, resentment, inferiority, lies, false pride, superiority, self-doubt, and ego do exist in the world, and they will go on existing long after I have left the earth. Just as equally so too will joy, peace, love, hope, serenity, humility, kindness, benevolence, empathy, generosity, truth, compassion, and faith.

Today, with a free and healthy mind, rather than be paralysed by that knowledge, I am at peace with it.

Every day, I do my best. And that is enough.

Fear Prevents Progress

Between stimulus and response there is a space. In that space is our power to choose our response. In our response lies our growth and our freedom.
~ Viktor Frankl

Possibly, the greatest and toughest thing you will ever learn (if you choose to learn) is that the things which happen to you do not cause your reaction.

Terrible, unspeakable things that should never have happened may have happened to you, and you have every right to blame, and yet when you blame, you give away your power.

It is not fair. But it is true.

When you blame, whether that blame be directed toward yourself, an illness, your brain, or another human being, for what you do or the way you are, you are giving away your one true power, the power to choose your response and your actions.

You have at any point in time an infinite number of ways in which you can choose to act, and whether you know this yet or not does not make it any less true.

The reality is… you are the only one who gets to decide which wolf you feed.

What is Recovered?

I am going to share with you briefly my definition of recovered. However, it is far more important that you come up with your own definition. I have worked with numerous people who've recovered from EDs, and definitions vary. Only you can decide what exactly it is that will be different in your life to let you know you've reached recovery.

I highly encourage you to take a moment to answer this question for yourself: What would make recovery "worth it" to me?

I can guarantee there will be bonuses you didn't see coming but it's useful to have a "why" to begin with.

Certainty

> *Please don't let your potential remain potential.*
> *~ Bonnie Killip*

To me, recovered means many things, all of which are difficult to capture in words but I will endeavour to give it a go. To me, recovered, more than anything, is a profound difference in how I feel now compared to when I lived with AN.

To me, recovered is the difference between living in fear, pain, and shame and living in love, clarity, and wisdom.

To me, recovered is when your mind is yours.

To me, recovered is when all those unobtainable possibilities and empty hopes that have been stuck in your mind become real choices.

If I had to name just one defining feature of recovery, it would be certainty. I now have certainty and confidence in myself. I now have a full and everlasting trust in my worth and in my ability to meet my needs. I now have a full and everlasting trust in my being a meaningful and valuable part of this world.

To me, recovered is having the kind of certainty that comes from not just understanding or knowing intellectually but wholeheartedly believing and feeling that I am enough.

There is no convincing, no arguing, and no incessant need to prove myself (to myself or to others). There is instead a constant and stable sense of peace and contentment with who I am, who I have been, and who I am becoming.

To me, recovered is a deep sense of self. This self is a person I am truly proud to be. I worked hard to become her.

There are and always will be things I can learn and expand upon, and I strive for growth and improving this world we call home each and every day, and I will do so for the rest of my life. Yet, at the same time, I know without question that at my core, at my most fundamental level, I am more than okay just as I am. I also know all the pain and suffering of the world is not mine alone to fix and that amidst the pain and suffering I can allow myself to live a life.

Recovered is Natural

To me, the most important thing about recovered is that it is natural. Recovered to me is when taking care of your body, mind, and soul come naturally. Recovered is no longer about fighting. Recovered is no longer about the incessant need to motivate yourself to avoid "bad" behaviours or to do "good" behaviours. Rather, it is finding yourself naturally seeking and enjoying behaviours that support your health and wellbeing.

Recovered is when you are doing the things which were once hard and no longer using the ED behaviours to cope, not because you have to force yourself not to or guilt or trick yourself into it but because you no longer feel the compulsion of the ED way of doing things.

You are appreciative of your life as an imperfectly perfect human being, and this is far more important to you than any identification with being sick, in recovery, or even brave or a warrior.

Contentment

God, grant me the serenity to accept the things I cannot change, the courage
to change the things I can,
and the wisdom to know the difference.
~ Reinhold Niebuhr

To me, recovered is being content with what is within and not within your control to change or influence.

When you accept that what you have control over is only a limited number of things, you have more time, energy, productivity, creativity, and happiness to direct into all those things which truly matter to you.

The less energy you spend on stress and trying to control other people and things outside your control the more energy you have for life.

Get Your Hopes Up (And Get Them Shattered!)

Recovered is sunshine and rainbows.
~ Bonnie Killip

People will tell you recovered is not sunshine and rainbows to keep you "realistic", with the noble intention of preventing you from getting your hopes up and being disappointed.

Adopt this outlook if you want, but I'd much sooner recommend getting your hopes up! I'd much more highly recommended you get every one of your hopes sky high, because you will never be disappointed with your recovered life.

You will still face struggles and challenges, you will still get hurt, experience pain, have bad days and hard experiences, but never, ever will you be disappointed that you reached full recovery.

I don't believe it's possible to recover and think, *Is this it? I'd rather go back to living with AN*. Have you ever heard someone who's recovered say they wished they'd not recovered or that they wished they'd waited longer or got a little sicker before they recovered?

It doesn't happen.

Those aren't the thoughts of a healthy and happy person, but they are common concerns when you're living with an ED. That maybe, somehow, you'll regret recovering.

There's a reason why no one regrets recovering, and that is when you are happily working with, rather than against, yourself, life truly is amazing.

What it is not is amazing because it is problem free.

Life is for getting your hopes up and getting them shattered, life is for going all in and getting your heart broken.

Because you can.

When you are well nourished and supporting your needs, you will be more than capable of competently overcoming all the challenges life will throw your way.

Imagine if you spent the rest of your life not getting your hopes up out of fear you'd be let down or get hurt?

Imagine flatlining through life… what a life that would be. Theoretically, you may prevent some pain, but you'd also prevent a lot more pleasure.

Allow yourself to get your hopes up.

Future healthy and happy you can handle it.

The Other Side of Sick

Recovery is not about pursing solely the cessation of symptoms. It is your chance to explore what you truly want instead.
~ Bonnie Killip

The goal of the life you will live on the other side of the ED is not a life simply with the absence of the ED.

Yes, you read that correctly. Maybe that's a new concept to you but it's true.

I know there was a point in time where my highest hope for my life was just to remain out of hospital for as long as possible.

To not die.

To be free of the ED would have been ideal (I didn't see that as possible though). Beyond that, I couldn't have described what it was I wanted.

The goal of the life you will live on the other side of the ED is a truly happy and fulfilling life. By your definition and your values. A life in which you belong and are fully immersed in doing other things; so much so that it would be a huge effort and inconvenience to go back to the ED way of doing things.

It is key that you hear this, because one of the biggest barriers to recovery can be the sense that because recovery is unspeakably painful, life will be no better on the other side. What you must understand is that this is not true.

When you are recovered, you no longer have to fight against the ED, because it is gone.

How Do I Know When I am Recovered?

This is a question I am asked frequently. The first response I wrote to this question was long, detailed, and very logically thought out, but the truth is much simpler, and it is this; you will know.

Oh gosh, you will know!

You will know when you are recovered, and it won't be because you can tick off a list of "yes, I do that's" or "no, I don't do that's anymore".

It will be a knowing in your heart with full and unquestionable certainty, and you will trust that knowing because you now trust yourself.

Perhaps the only true sign that you are recovered is that you will no longer feel a need to ask the question "how do I know when I am recovered?"

What is Recovery?

Recovery is about relinquishing the need to know ahead of time those things you cannot know ahead of time.
~ Bonnie Killip

Recovery is a journey. A journey with a purpose but a journey first and foremost.

Recovery is all the things that you must learn in order to know, respect, and love yourself, to ultimately become the person capable of living the life you want.

Recovery, more than being a one-off monumental feat, is the less than glamorous extra spoon of ice-cream through the tears, it is eating the muesli bar when there's no one to tell you it's the right thing to do, it is setting your alarm to eat a morning snack, and it is not going for that run when it would be so easy and feel much better if you did.

Recovery takes doing the things when you are terrified.

Recovery takes doing the things when you are worn out, full, and disinterested.

Updating Your Mind

When it feels disheartening to learn that trauma changes the brain, remember that healing changes the brain too.
~ Tyndal Schreiner

Recovery is learning who you are underneath all the restrictions imposed on you by the ED, family, friends, school, society, social media, or others, because under all this, you are your own phenomenal and unique person.

Recovery is about learning who you are.

Recovery is leaning to trust yourself to live as you.

Recovery is a process, because you've lived with an illness for I don't know how long but long enough that it has changed the structure and function of your brain.

That's profound.

Yet in no way does it mean this change is locked in and the illness is your destiny. In fact, it means the opposite.

We know much about neuroscience, we know much about EDs, and though by no means do we know it all, we know enough to know your brain is changeable.

AN does not need to be your life story.

The very fact that your brain changed to accommodate the illness is proof that your brain *can* change. Your brain can change to update and create new neuronal patterns and pathways to get rid of the illness and put amazing things in its place.

It takes work to undo (just as it took work to get into and is taking work to maintain) but it is by no means work that is beyond you.

How Long Does Recovery Take?

> *Knowing how doesn't mean anything until you do it.*
> *~ Bonnie Killip*

Do you feel the desire to "take it slow" in recovery?

It is now inconceivable to me that taking it slow was something I wanted to do. Even alone and terrified in a hospital bed over a thousand kilometres away from home, I wanted to take it slow.

In hindsight, I understand that it was simply my inability to trust that I was doing the right thing, my need to have more information, or my disbelief that recovered was possible or would be any better. I wanted to have it all figured out and know exactly how things would go in order to put in one hundred percent effort.

I now see I wasn't taking it slow; I simply wasn't recovering.

I was one foot in and one foot out even when my body was shutting down.

There is no logical reason to get better slowly.

If you put yourself in the shoes of a healthy, thriving person joyously engaged and fulfilled in daily life, would putting your health and life on the line by prolonging your recovery make sense?

No. Not even slightly. Especially when the alternative is getting better quickly and experiencing health, happiness, connection, and contributing to this wonderful world sooner.

You now recognise that you want recovery, so why prolong the pain of getting there? If you are going to recover one day (and if you've come this far through this book, I can be certain you very much plan to), why waste time stretching out the inevitable?

Wanting to recover slowly is like wanting to get better from a cold slowly or wanting to recover from cancer gradually rather than immediately… It simply isn't logical.

Getting better slowly is a perpetuation of the illness.

Two Areas to Address When Making Change

I haven't failed a thousand times, I've just found a thousand ways not to make a lightbulb.
~ Thomas Edison

If you feel there is a benefit to holding on, getting better slowly or when you are ready, consider asking yourself if either of these apply to you:

1. You feel afraid.

    and

2. You don't know how.

These are the two reasons we (collectively as human beings) struggle with when it comes to making change. Choose which one it is for you (it can be a combination) and get the help to work on it (them) now so they no longer exist.

The following model of recovery is my offering of how you may be able to practically achieve this.

3.2 Introduction to the Two Major Stages of Recovery

Experience is simply the name we give our mistakes.
~ Oscar Wilde

After attempting recovery more times than I care to count, I can, in retrospect, identify two distinct stages or phases of the recovery journey, characterised by shifts in psychological and physiological needs, and within each of those two phases, there are in total three components that need to be addressed in order for recovery to be complete:

Introduction to The Two-Stages Model of Recovery

What if it were all so much simpler than you have imagined?...
~ Bonnie

Surrender

1. Weight Gain
2. Repair of Physical Damage

Growth

3. Psychological Development

Why the Two-Stages Model?

If a man knows not to which port he sails, no wind is favourable.
~ Seneca

I know that perhaps seeing recovery put into such a simplified model may feel inspiring, or perhaps it may feel insulting.

I don't mean for this simplification to imply that it is easy to reach any of these stages. Remember, I am not saying, "you should do this" or "why don't you just do that?" without ever having been in the hot seat. I am someone who's been very much in the hot seat.

It is for exactly this reason that I am simplifying it.

It is my belief that simplifying recovery and having tangible milestones (and a clear plan on how to reach them) makes the otherwise incredibly daunting and overwhelming task of recovery achievable.

When you know what you are aiming for, you can see that each choice you make has the potential to either draw you closer to or take you further away from the target.

Each choice you make is casting a vote for your future.

The Three-Component Model of Recovery

Let's now take a look at each of the two components of recovery in more detail, because it is within these seemingly little components that the entire journey from illness to health is found. It is your variation of this journey which you must undertake in order to reach leadership of your life (otherwise known as recovered) beginning with:

Stage One of Recovery: Surrender

Often, we tell ourselves, "Don't just sit there, do something!" But when we practice awareness, we discover something unusual. We discover that the opposite may be more helpful: "Don't just do something, sit there!"
~ Nhat Hanh

Component 1 and 2 - Weight Gain & Repair of Physical Damage

The first stage of recovery is about giving up the fight. It's about letting go. It is the ultimate surrender, and is comprised of two components:

1. Weight gain

and

2. Repair of physical damage.

Letting Go to Gain Everything

> *Well done is better than well said.*
> *~ Benjamin Franklin*

This stage of recovery is not about having all the answers to your problems (if you had the answers, you wouldn't have the problems…). Instead, it is about relinquishing the (perceived) control. It is about trusting in others.

If you're thinking that's a strange thing for me to say after pages and pages about how recovered is a life where you have certainty and control, freedom and autonomy you're right; however, recovery is not recovered.

Recovery is the journey to recovered, and, paradoxically, in order to gain leadership of your life later, you must first let go now. Later, you will learn how to take control and responsibility of your actions and learn to choose your thoughts and what you want in your life, but in the beginning, during stage One, it is about letting go. It is about surrendering, because it is only when you surrender to what is, instead of what "should" be, that you open space in which to become you. Something you can't hope to do while you're "trying" to be you before you are you.

There are a lot of people out there doing the recommended motions of recovery because they feel they "should" want to but feeling you should want to is monumentally different to wanting to. If there's a part of you that doesn't really want to recover, that's okay. Rather than fighting with it or trying to convince it, surrender and give the part that does want to recover a chance.

Sometimes It Starts with Breakfast

I know for me there when moments where relinquishing control was a relief. There when moments I sobbed with gratitude. Especially during those first few days post hospitalisation when I stayed with my parents and I would wake up knowing I could eat breakfast. I cried silently as I lay in bed, bathed in the absurdly calm early morning silence that followed weeks of ceaseless beeps, harsh voices, and fluorescent hospital lighting.

To know that I didn't have to battle within myself over what and when and how and where to eat because my mum was going to make breakfast for me was incredible.

And yet, at the same time, it was utterly terrifying, because of course the contradiction was that in no way did I want to actually eat the breakfast.

In the back of my mind, I knew the "permission" to eat was finite.

Trusting Despite, Not Because

This is the absurdity of recovery: you will feel everything at once and nothing at all. This is why recovery is a commitment and not a one-off choice.

Recovery is not about learning to control the fear that comes with the loss of control, nor is it about knowing how it will all turn out before giving it a go. Recovery is about giving it a go despite the fear. Recovery is about giving it a go when you don't have the answers and you don't know that it is going to work out okay.

You Can Be Both at The Same Time

It's okay to be both terrified and excited. It's okay to both want recovery and want the "safety" and familiarity of the ED. You can have more than one feeling at the same time and still choose recovery, because successful recovery does not necessitate being completely motivated a hundred percent of the time.

The Best Thing in Early Recovery is for it to Be Out of Your Hands

If you're in the early stages of recovery from AN, you're not in an ideal position to be making the decisions you need to make (even if you think you are).

If you can let it go.

Seek great help and keep in the forefront of your mind that the help you receive is from a person or people you have chosen, and they are therefore people you trust. Work with them and trust their guidance, even if it scares you.

Remember always—recovery is your choice.

To surrender to others is also not a permanent solution, because the second stage of recovery is where you get to explore and experiment, but this must be when you want to and not just because you feel you should. Which means you can't get there without first going through this first component of surrender, where you accept that you can't do it all alone.

We're now going to look more deeply at the two components within this first stage of recovery, "Surrender," with the intention of offering guidance on where to focus your time and energy, beginning with:

Component One. Weight Gain

I never dreamed about success, I worked for it.
~ Estee Lauder

Introduction to Weight Gain

In reality, weight gain is simply a part of component of two (repair of physical damage) and 3 (psychological development) and not a separate component on its own, but as weight gain is easily measurable, is a well-known component of recovery from AN and can be used somewhat as an indicator for repair of physical damage, I have included it as a separate component.

I also like to be upfront and honest, and the fact is if treatment, recovery, and health were possible at a low body weight, we'd do that, but it's just not possible. It is a universal truth that there is no health to be found in being "underweight". If you are underweight or if your body is in starvation, then there's no avoiding it; weight gain is a necessary part of your recovery, and even if you are not underweight in order to repair your relationship with food and your body, it may still be necessary that you gain weight.

Weight Gain Vs Weight Restoration

I use the phrase "weight gain" rather than "weight restoration", as is commonly used, for the reason that restoration implies you are returning to some former fixed and decided weight. Which is just not the case. This is not the case for several reasons, including the fact that the most common time to develop an ED is the early teenage years. Meaning, if you are in recovery years later as an adult, the weight you were before the ED became a part of your life will not be your healthy weight now.

In any instance, it is common for weight gain to initially go beyond what's referred to as your "set point" weight or your "ideal" healthy weight (or what I like to call your "happy weight") and then drop down later when your body trusts it is not going to be starved again any time soon.

This "overshoot" is not unique to ED recovery but a general pattern observed in those who go through periods of starvation (due to any cause, be that experimental, illness, war, or famine) followed by subsequent refeeding. What this means is that if somehow you did theoretically know what your healthiest weight would be if you were to aim for this, you're likely aiming too low initially.

The other thing to know is that the initial distribution of weight will likely be different than after full, long-term recovery, because fat stores are the first to replenish.

Only after fat stores are replenished and returned to pre starvation levels or higher will the composition of the rest of your body begin to change (i.e. increases in muscle mass and redistribution of fat), which equates to further changes in weight.

On top of this, the definition of recovery is letting go of the need for unrealistic levels of control, and what you weigh falls firmly within this category. Recovery means gaining weight to where your body wants to sit naturally, without any form of restriction, and that can't be pre-decided. Not you, your doctor, your dietitian, the BMI calculation, nor any other tool or person knows what this point is. We can do our best to estimate, but at the end of the day, only your body knows.

You Must Eat

A crucial part of recovery is nutritionally supporting your body and brain. Food is the means by which we do this.

In other words, you must eat.

Weight gain and food are not the be all and end all of recovery, but in order to be capable of adequately dealing with the underlying "problems", it is without question necessary to have a functioning brain.

More importantly than having a functioning brain to do the work necessary to recover from AN, an adequately functioning brain is necessary to live the rest of your life anywhere near the top of your game. A healthy brain is needed to live the rest of your life present and well fuelled, to enjoy all the moments you get the opportunity to experience. Isn't that the whole point of life—to be in it while you're in it?

You Can Think, Feel, and Live Only Because You Eat

At the structural level, changing and updating your neurology takes energy. At the functional level, your brain literally runs off sugar and fat. That means you can think at all only because you eat. Your brain therefore is always going to be limited in function by how well you eat.

No Amount of Therapy Can Compensate for a Nutritional Lack

In some cases, depression, obsessional thinking, anxiety, obsessive compulsive behaviours, cognitive impairment, slowed thought processing, impaired short-term memory, reduced cognitive flexibility and concentration, attention difficulties, and other psychiatric symptoms can represent the reversible or at least partly reversible effects starvation has on the brain[59,60].

If nutritional nourishment stays forever a limiting factor, it doesn't matter how much therapy you attend or the depth of your learning, knowledge, and insight of what to do; you fundamentally won't be able to make the changes you want.

If your brain is not functioning properly, no amount of therapy will be of lasting help, because no amount of therapy can fix a nutritional lack.

At the end of the day, you are a biological being, and as such, limited by your biology.

The Hardware and Software of Your Brain

For a moment, I want you to think of your brain as if it is a computer. There are two fundamental components which make up computers, allowing them to be as useful as they are. There's the hardware, which is the physical stuff that makes up a computer, and the software, which are the programs you use on the computer.

Just as you would not be able to run some of the fast software programs of today on the old hardware of the computers of the past, the same is true of your brain.

If you're trying to get a malnourished and starved brain that doesn't have access to its total capacity to run a brand new and updated program far beyond its development, it's simply not possible.

The flip side of this is also true in that you can have the most well-tuned, nutritionally supported brain in the world, but if you're running outdated or faulty software, you're also not going to be making full use of your brain's capabilities.

Feed your brain well so that your hardware is state of the art. Combine this with updating your skills and resources so you are running great software that is based on the life you live now and not through past. Then you will live an amazing life.

Choosing to Eat is Never the Wrong Decision

Food is the foundation of every human being's life. Food gives us energy and passion, and the more nutrition your brain and body have the more capable, resourceful, and successful you will be.

Once you get past eating simply to survive, what you eat takes on a whole new role, for what you now choose to eat allows you to thrive.

Good nutrition is a necessity for those who want to go far. If you cannot remember anything else in the moments your emotions, confusion, and overwhelm take over and you start to find the decision over whether or not to eat or what to eat debilitating, remember this: choosing to eat is never, ever the wrong decision.

Unconditional Eating

Don't fall into the trap of needing to have all your problems sorted and then you can eat, because some problems you won't be able to sort until you are nourished, some problems will be a lot easier to sort when you are nourished, some problems you'll simply have to live with but be able to cope with better when you're nourished, and some problems will simply go away when you are nourished.

Combine renourishment and addressing the underlying "problems" and you have inevitable success.

Just Because You Want it Doesn't Mean it's Easy

I despised being underweight. I thought I looked disgusting. I avoided going out because I was ashamed of the way I looked. I avoided mirrors for years. I desperately wanted a belly and boobs like my friends. There was no moment where I strived for weight loss or thought looking skeletal was attractive.

The point I am trying to make is that you must recognise that no matter how much you consciously want it, weight gain will be a challenge, and you know what? You're allowed to both want it and fear it at the same time. That's the game of recovery. Which wolf will you feed?

Relinquish the Need for it to Be Logical

Would you be prepared to give up the need for a logical explanation as to why you are afraid of food, of why you're thinking, feeling, and doing the weird things you are?

Because at the end of the day, it doesn't matter. You don't need to understand *why* in order to change.

AN is an illness. An illness in which fear of food is one of the distinguishing features, and that, by definition, makes weight gain hard.

Surrender the need to analyse, judge, or search for meaning. The meaning will come. I promise, in hindsight, you will understand, but not before you've done the doing. The learning comes before the understanding, and the learning is not a spectator sport.

The Physical Challenges of Weight Gain

Weight gain in recovery is not only mentally challenging but also physically challenging. Physically, your gastrointestinal tract (GI) will have suffered, and therefore your digestion will be compromised. Which means there is a very high chance you will experience ongoing bloating, fullness, pain, nausea, diarrhoea, and constipation, as well as a whole list of other uncomfortable symptoms.

While knowing this doesn't make it easier or lessen the anguish, I want you to know that it is all a normal part of renourishment, and there is only one thing which lessens it: consistent and adequate nourishment[56,57]. With consistent and adequate nourishment, all the damage and the symptoms the damages are causing are reversible and repairable.

Honestly, if you get all this nutrition stuff worked out right now, you may be able to live a future healthier than if you'd never fallen sick. In some ways, you're in a better position than many others to turn your health and life around.

It's not too late.

And if not in any case it's still going to be a better option for your future to heal than to go on suffering.

The Symptoms Won't Go Before the Damage is Repaired

If you don't eat because of the distress these GI symptoms cause, you might alleviate them or avoid them in that moment, but please know this is very different from fixing them.

Continuing to eat despite these symptoms is the only way you will gain sustained (lifelong) relief from them, because eating is the only way the damage the symptoms are a result of can be repaired.

Climb Aboard the Metabolic Rollercoaster

Changes in your metabolism as your body comes out of starvation and malnutrition can also make weight gain difficult.

To begin with, you may find you gain weight relatively quickly, and then it may slow, or you may find that you begin to lose weight even while keeping to the same amount of food which once helped you gain weight.

This is because you will require increasing amounts of food to maintain and gain weight, for reasons I will briefly touch on now and further expand on in the second component of the Two-Stage Model of Recovery (Repair of Physical Damage).

First Quick

When your body is in starvation, your metabolism slows to decrease your body's overall use of fuel. Therefore, when you begin to eat more and have an energy intake above what you were eating during restriction, you may initially gain weight relatively quickly. This initial ease of weight gain can often cause a fear response that your body can't be trusted and that you will continue to gain weight forever or that you may lose the help and support you need when you no longer "look sick" or even that you're doing something "wrong".

As a result of these very real feeling fears, there can be a consequent unintentional decrease in food intake, essentially perpetuating the problem by putting your body and metabolic processes back into starvation mode.

Water Weight

In addition to your slowed metabolism, some of the initial quick weight gain will be water as you become rehydrated. People with AN are commonly dehydrated (I'm not necessarily using the correct technical term here, but it helps as a descriptor), and this isn't usually from not drinking enough water but from not eating enough carbohydrates.

When you haven't eaten enough carbohydrates and your stores of glycogen are depleted (quick reminder: glycogen is the storage form of glucose in your muscles and liver, glucose being the molecules carbohydrates are broken down into within your digestive tract. Glucose being your brain and most of your body's preferred fuel source), you will be dehydrated because glycogen is stored with water in a 1:3 ratio. What this means is that for every gram of glycogen stored in your liver and muscles 3-4 grams of water are also stored alongside. At full storage capacity, it is estimated that the human body can store up to six hundred grams of glycogen, which equates to 2.4L-3L of water, which is 2.4-3kg of water.

Therefore, you can see that a quick weight gain of 3-3.6kg (water plus glycogen stores being replenished) in the early stages of refeeding is purely attributed to water weight (plus glycogen).

Not fat, not muscle; just water and glycogen.

What this also means is that while this initial quick weight gain is important in rehydration and setting your body up to begin repair, it's not necessarily indicative of any repair per se.

Fat Weight

Following a period of starvation and the reintroduction of adequate food, fat is the first tissue to be stored.

It appears the human body likes to bring fat stores back to or above pre weight loss levels before any fat free mass (i.e. muscle) is repaired. Which, from your body's perspective, storing fat as a priority over muscle gain makes perfect sense, because if you were to enter starvation again, your body can use these fat stores as fuel.

The replenishment of fat stores as priority further contributes to weight gain being more rapid in the early stages of renourishment, because your body is able to make and store fat quicker than it is able to make muscle.

Another thing to be aware of is that the gain of fat tissue is generally not uniform across your body. The pattern of fat gain that is generally experienced is an accumulation around your belly and triceps[58] until stores are fully replenished.

Then, if, and only if, adequate nutrition continues to be supplied for a continuous period of time without prolonged interruption with restrictive periods, will this fat redistribute and possibly decrease as fat free mass (including muscle) is synthesised.

Then Slow

To restore your functioning metabolism and health, you need to continue to eat. After this quick initial weight gain due to the three factors explained above (slowed metabolism, water weight, and fat weight), your metabolism will then speed up.

As you continue to provide your body with adequate and consistent nutrition, your body begins to trust that there is abundant food in the environment and there is no need to hold onto everything. This gives your metabolism permission to kick up, and by kick up, I mean it really can go sky high.

There are several reasons for this increase in metabolism, which really was a huge factor for me personally and made weight gain past a certain point feel impossible.

I will go into more detail about why an increase in metabolism makes weight gain hard in the "Extreme Hunger" section under the third component within the Two Stage Model of Recovery (repair of physical damage). For now, we'll stick to the psychology of how this feels and what you need to know.

You Are Different

This increase in metabolism is one of the reasons it is important during recovery to relinquish comparing your food intake to others.

The food you need in order to recover from starvation, malnutrition, and to gain weight is substantially more than what someone who has not been in starvation would need to eat to achieve the same weight gain. It is more than you would need to eat had you not gone through this experience.

Fact: The moment you compare or try to copy what others are eating, you will lose weight.

I was obsessed with "fitting in", of copying others of believing they must be doing it more correct than me. There was also not a single time where it did not result in weight loss and disaster.

It doesn't matter what other people eat. What other people eat truly has nothing to do with what you need to eat, not just in recovery but ever. It is only what you eat which has the ability to support or limit your health, happiness, and fulfillment.

If that's hard for you to feel now, know that you don't have to be there yet, because you'll get there. For now, understand that you are in a different position. Your body needs lots of nourishing food in order to be able to move beyond weight gain and onto repairing the physical damage done during starvation and malnutrition. This repair requires consistent effort.

The goal of eating in recovery is not mindful or intuitive eating. The goal of eating in recovery is not even "normal" eating. It's eating when you're not hungry, it's eating when no one else is eating, it's eating by the clock, it's eating things you're not even sure you like or wouldn't be your preference and it's eating when you're bloated, full, and uncomfortable.

"Normal" eating comes later.

Summary to Component One. Weight Gain

In summary, weight gain during recovery is necessary for the healing and development of your body, brain, and mind in order to not only survive this illness and get out of a life that's harming you but most importantly to begin to create and to live the life you want.

Let us now look at what is involved in the second component of stage 1 of the Three-Component Model of Recovery.

Component Two. Repair of Physical Damage

Today you have a hundred percent of your life left.
~ Tom Landry

Introduction to Repair of Physical Damage

Repair of physical damage is the reversal of the damage starvation and malnutrition have done to your body. This is irrespective of the amount of weight you lost or what you weigh now.

Even if you are not "underweight" or have regained weight to a "healthy weight", as deemed by any outside measure, the reality is your body has been through extreme stress, and repairing this internal damage requires nourishment (otherwise known as food).

Malnutrition is Not "Done" When You are Weight Restored

Repairing physical damage requires energy above what gaining weight requires.

It may take months and more likely years for your body to completely recover and replenish.

Studies have shown an elevated metabolism can persist six to twelve months or longer after a healthy weight has been reached and regular and adequate nutrition established, and there are other studies indicating metabolism may be altered for life.

I once truly believed that my metabolism was altered for life, because it really did not appear to matter how much I ate or for how long, I felt I could not gain weight or when I did I was unable to maintain it.

I was constantly accused of hiding food, not eating what I was saying I was eating, exercising, vomiting, using laxatives, and so on when I wasn't, so extreme (or rather "normal" in the case of recovering from AN as I was to find out years later through my own research) was my experience with hypermetabolism.

However, I now believe it's possible to restore a normal metabolism. It is done through a period of overeating, and by this I mean going beyond the conservative confines of any meal plan.

It is my theory, and my experience, which happens to be in line with the experiences of others who've recovered from AN, that in order to truly allow your body to come out of all these weird, altered states, it takes a feast.

It takes a period of sustained high, uncontrolled energy intake, and it seems that this indicates to your body not only that the famine is over but that the food supply is now more than adequate.

What this all means is that even if you or your loved one has gained weight, are within a healthy weight range, are eating adequate and regular meals, your/their metabolism may still be elevated and they can't go back to eating a "regular" diet now that they are at a "healthy" weight because a regular diet wouldn't be enough (and by a "regular" diet I mean what would otherwise have been enough had you or they not gone through this experience).

While we may be built to withstand starvation in that we can endure and survive it, we aren't built to bounce back and thrive the instant we get adequate food, especially if the undernourishment has been prolonged.

It is not a small thing your body has been and is going through; respect that. Malnutrition is not "done" when you are weight restored.

Your Nutritional Requirements Don't Decrease Because You've Gained Weight

Your weight is an indicator of health but not the most reliable one.

Your body is still fighting hard to repair, and your high metabolism will persist until all damage is repaired. I know it is difficult to continue to eat far above what others around you are eating, especially when you have reached a "healthy" weight, because it doesn't seem to make sense, but I assure you, and I hope you are beginning to see, that it does make sense.

As bizarre and incomprehensible as it may sound to you now, you really will know when you are truly ready to eat less.

What your body needs is not something you can choose, force, control, or base off what any research or anyone else is doing. If you are attempting to do so even with the best of health intentions, let that be your clear sign you're not there yet, because when you are there, you won't feel the need to judge your food intake.

You'd be forgiven for thinking otherwise with the overwhelming emphasis Western culture places on how to "eat less", but the truth is the human body takes a lot of fuel to run, even if we are to put recovery aside for a moment.

Additionally, studies are showing now that people genetically predisposed to AN have genes linked to altered metabolism, meaning their bodies simply react differently to food intake and may naturally require higher levels of nutrition, be this overall energy intake and/or particular micronutrients.

In any case, undernourishment is irrefutably a trigger for developing and perpetuating AN. Therefore, if you're finding yourself in quasi recovery, that is somewhat there but you know you're not where you want to be, you need to eat more (yes, including even if you're already eating quadruple those around you).

Your body needs what your body needs.

Some Realities of Emerging from Hell

If you are entering recovery from AN, the reality is your body has been through hell and there are some things it still must go through to readjust as you begin to care for and nourish yourself.

In the remainder of this section on Stage Two of Recovery "Repair of Physical Damage", I am going to describe a few things you may experience during the recovery process, because while the physical need for weight restoration is well known and you are generally prepared for that one, there are a bunch of other (spoiler alert; mostly unpleasant) physical changes no one tells you about that also may present themselves.

It is my intention that through describing some of the things you may experience as your body goes about repairing the damage, you will gain reassurance that you are on the right path. Consider taking it as a reminder to not back down when they happen and most of all to give loving your body through them a go.

It's easy for me to say things like "love your body" now, but it wasn't always, and I know it might make you flinch to read those words. I know if I had read them back when I was going through this, I'd have probably skipped the next few pages, maybe even threw away such an absurd book immediately! Please don't do that, because the information that follows may be the thing that gets you through. That little "love your body" remark is there as a challenge and to show you the transformational mindset you are on your way to brining into existence.

Welcome to the Jungle

The harsh reality of choosing recovery and allowing your body to heal is that you may experience any or all the following:

Refeeding & Refeeding Syndrome

Refeeding is the name we give to the process of reintroducing food following a period of eating food below your body's requirements for energy and nutrients.

During the early stages of refeeding, there is the risk for a potentially life-threatening condition called refeeding syndrome. Refeeding syndrome is your body's response to abruptly receiving nutrition above what it has adapted to. This fast change in nutritional intake disrupts the electrolyte balance of your body's fluid compartments (your blood and the fluid between your cells). The electrolyte disturbance is due to a switch from fasting gluconeogenesis (the glucose your body needs to survive being synthesised from lactate, pyruvate, glycerol, and amino acids ie not directly from the carbohydrates you are eating) to carbohydrate-induced insulin release (insulin being released in response to eating carbohydrates), which triggers rapid uptake of potassium, phosphate, and magnesium into your cells to metabolise the increased intake of carbohydrates[61].

You don't need to understand all that is happening to know refeeding syndrome can have a number of harmful outcomes, including convulsions, delirium, brain damage, hypotension, kidney failure, heart failure, and death.

Because refeeding syndrome is serious, there are guidelines on the "appropriate" rate to reintroduce calories (food), especially carbohydrates, back into the diet of someone who has not been eating adequately with the aim of reducing the risk for developing refeeding syndrome. To give you an idea of these guidelines they generally start with incrementally increasing kilojoule/calorie intake over the course of a few days to two weeks, along with daily B vitamin supplementation and electrolyte restoration as necessary.

B vitamins (in particular vitamin B1 or thiamine) are necessary because these vitamins help your body to process carbohydrates. People with AN who are at risk of refeeding syndrome are malnourished and are therefore likely deficient in B vitamins and unable to adequately process (metabolise) carbohydrates without the supplemented B vitamins. This is why the supplementation is necessary.

There is not a great deal of evidence to support the use of refeeding guidelines in patients in recovery from AN, and many see refeeding guidelines as being too conservative and placing patients at even higher risk of 'underfeeding syndrome', exacerbating malnourishment and further deterioration. For this reason, many hospitals are beginning to or have removed refeeding guidelines from their ED treatment protocol.

The hospitals in which I have worked (and been a patient) still use refeeding guidelines, but this is now more as a cautionary rather than as a strictly evidence-based tool.

In any case, it is important to have your blood monitored regularly to identify and minimise your risk of the disastrous effects of refeeding syndrome as you go through the process of refeeding. I don't recommend doing recovery alone for more reasons than refeeding syndrome but it is another reason to add to the list.

During refeeding, as you continue to eat adequately and regularly, your body will come out of starvation, and your reduced metabolism (hypometabolism) will amp up. This is when you may experience something I introduced briefly earlier on in this section. What is commonly referred to as extreme hunger (or hypermetabolism).

Extreme Hunger (Hypermetabolism)

Extreme hunger is exactly what the name implies—the experience of having an insatiable appetite.

If you are experiencing extreme hunger, or when you do, please know that it is "normal". That is; it is normal in recovery, it's not normal to everyday life after recovery or for people who haven't gone through starvation, but for where you are and with all the abnormal things your body has gone through, it is your normal.

Extreme hunger is different to experiencing variations in daily hunger levels (i.e., being hungrier some days and less hungry others, which you will experience after recovery). Extreme hunger feels like you have an unquenchable appetite and there is often a compulsion to eat even when you are physically and often painfully full.

Why Does Extreme Hunger Occur?

Extreme hunger occurs as a natural response of your body to having been stared. It is your body furiously trying to meet the huge energy costs of repairing the damage done during starvation and malnutrition. Your body is trying to repair the damage and restore your health as quickly as possible, and the more food it gets, the quicker it can do this.

Physical and Psychological Torment
Going from an underactive metabolism where you were able to survive off very little a day to an overactive metabolism can feel scary and overwhelming.

I am lost for words with how to describe the utter physical and psychological torment this inflicted (made worse by the fact that like everything during recovery, I kept it to myself because I was deeply ashamed).

I felt completely out of control. I felt like a monster.

My belly would be full beyond capacity, constantly popping out like a bloated round, tight, beach ball, and I would still be hungry.

I would dread finishing eating, and when I did finish eating, I'd count the hours until I could eat again. Making it from breakfast to morning tea was too long, and I'd have to have a snack between.

Extreme Hunger is a Normal Biological Response to Starvation

When you eat to this extreme hunger, you may find yourself in pain physically and most definitely mentally.

My best suggestion is to let go of the self-judgement.

Extreme hunger is not a flaw in your character, morals, or self-control, it's not personal, and it's not even unique to you. Extreme hunger is a normal biological response following a period of restriction, and your hunger will settle down, but not before the damage has been repaired.

If you are voraciously hungry, don't try to fight this; instead, eat to this, because it is exactly what your body is asking for, and your body is not asking for it for no reason. Your body is asking for it because it needs it. You need to eat more than people who are not in recovery.

The only way for extreme hunger to settle down permanently and restore your natural metabolism is to keep going and not go back to restriction. Going back to restriction to avoid extreme hunger will lead to your metabolism slowing down again, and all that means is you will just have to go through extreme hunger again. If you want to fully recover that is.

A Phenomenal Combination

Every time I started into a new "recovery" and attempt at weight restoration, I was determined to win. I was determined that this time I would beat anorexia once and for all. I was determined, and I was hungry. It was a phenomenal combination.

When I gave myself permission and a purpose to eat, I was ravenous. I was ravenous and I was on a mission. In this mode, I was unstoppable.

For a time.

As I gained weight and began to look and feel healthier and more capable, it scared me.

What was next?

I didn't know…

I became far less confident and certain because I still didn't know what I wanted outside of gaining weight.

There is No Way to Do Eating "Wrong"

I would often try to get someone else to be in charge of my food and mealtimes because eating to my hunger simply wasn't possible and I was afraid of myself if I tried to do it. I didn't trust myself if I was left to my own devices. I thought I'd never stop eating. I didn't know how much to eat, and it seemed like something I could get wrong. And getting it wrong felt worse than death.

Now it means nothing because there is no way a human being can get eating "wrong".

Strangely, the reality was the opposite of what the fear part of me was screaming at me anyway. Instead of overeating, when I was left to my own devices, the emptiness, the lack of self and purpose, the confusion, stress, and overwhelm took over, and I couldn't eat.

I would inevitably relapse, having no understanding why.

I'd followed the instructions of how to recover to a T. I'd done what everyone said I should do. I'd done what all the textbooks, doctors, dietitians, psychologists, and psychiatrists told me to do. I'd gained weight.

But I was more lost than ever.

Extreme Hunger and Socialising

Extreme hunger can feel overwhelming, especially, I found, when I was around other people.

Exposure to what others were eating or talking about what they were eating and knowing what I was eating was excruciating. I felt humiliated. I felt abnormal and ashamed of myself.

I felt like I was eating four to five times what anyone else I knew was eating, and still in my heart of hearts I felt like I needed more.

When I lived with AN, the comments others made about food impacted me greatly, and never in a positive way. I was deeply ashamed of eating, of the judgement of others, of breathing, of being seen, of taking up space, of everything, really. And because I had no sense of self, no filter or boundaries protecting me from what people said and did and what I took on board, I took it all on.

My mind fixated on things, twisted them, and interpreted them in disordered ways I can't fully describe now because it's impossible for me to connect to how that felt. But I felt it all so deeply. I had no other option.

I can honestly say that many of my relapses stemmed from some relatively benign comment someone made about my body or food or their own body or their own food. I had zero capacity to choose to not twist it through the ED lens and take it to heart.

They Don't Know

If people are commenting on your food during recovery (and I can guarantee they will), keep in your mind that they simply don't know. They haven't read this book, they aren't recovering from AN, and they are likely speaking from a place of good intentions, or at least a place where it means nothing to them.

I know and you know that it feels like they are attacking you, and even when you "know" they don't mean it the way you are taking it, I know that doesn't stop the barrage of emotions.

I assure you, on the other side of recovery, what anyone else says or does around food won't affect your ability to eat or your perception of self-worth. In fact, it won't affect a moment of your day because it won't matter to you. You will no longer have to try to not care or try to pretend their words and actions don't hurt, because they won't.

In recovery, there is no more "trying" and "pretending". There is only truth and peace. If you are planning on not caring what others say or eat one day, why let it affect you now? Why not make that one day today? Why not practice not letting the comments of others derail your path?

Do What is Within Your Power

While you can't avoid every situation where someone might comment on your food, this is not the goal. The goal is to be unaffected by such comments. However, before you're at that stage, there might be some people or situations in your life whom you could choose to not eat around for a while if they are truly triggering for you and impacting your recovery.

Consider making your recovery your priority.

If you constantly find yourself being triggered by one person or a few people in particular, and it is hindering your progress and even after you have spoken with them about it, they don't understand or make an attempt to change their actions or words, then you need to recognise and distance yourself from that.

It might be beyond their capability, and that's okay.

This is only a temporary tactic, because with the right help, you will develop your sense of self and won't be affected by what people say or do, but eating in the early stages of recovery is highly emotional.

You don't need to push yourself to do anything above the level you're at.

When you are recovered, I promise you that taking responsibility for your food won't be overwhelming. It will just be a part of life.

Happy for a Day or Happy for a Lifetime

Do you want to feel happy for a day or happy for a lifetime? Feeling happy for a lifetime requires of you in this moment to eat lots of food. Feeling happy for a lifetime requires of you in this moment to eat lots of high energy, nourishing, life promoting, life enabling, life enhancing food.

You don't have to love it or even enjoy it. You just have to do it.

Night Sweats

A common experience for people in recovery from AN is to wake up in the night drenched in sweat.

Night sweats typically occur in the early stages of refeeding, because when you are in the early stages of refeeding, you are extremely energy inefficient, and a disproportionately high percentage of your energy intake goes toward heat generation.

There's evidence to suggest hormonal changes also contribute to night sweats, but whatever the reasons, night sweats are not fun, and it's good to be prepared in the knowledge that this may happen, because the sweating is excessive. You and your sheets will be soaking wet.

Night sweats are a "normal" part of recovery, and these episodes will eventually pass as you continue to eat and your metabolism and hormones work themselves out.

Low Blood Glucose

Low BGLs are a risk during illness and still a risk during recovery, even when you are eating well, because of hypermetabolism (increased metabolism).

When you are hypermetabolic, your body is burning through everything you give it incredibly fast, making it hard to keep up with and easy to underestimate your needs.

Low BGLs are a concern because if you are awake and your BGLs drop, you can pass out and hit your head and risk concussion. On the other hand, if your BGLs drop while you're asleep, you risk going into a coma.

The only way to correct low BGLs is to eat more. In particular, carbohydrate rich foods, because glucose is the end breakdown product of carbohydrates. Carbohydrates include any of the grains (for example bread, rice, pasta, quinoa, oats), milk, starchy vegetables (potato, sweet potato, and corn), and fruits. It's useful to combine these carbohydrates with a source of protein and/or fat because this will slow their digestion and absorption, which helps keep your BGLs stable for a longer period of time.

I recommend having a snack before bed such as a mug of warm milk or hot chocolate with some biscuits, a smoothie containing peanut butter or other nut butter, and a piece of cake, toast, or a crumpet with yoghurt or cheese to keep your BGLs up overnight.

Even this may not always be enough, and some people find they have to have snacks through the night.

I would wake up at two a.m. religiously, drenched in sweat, not knowing what was going on, because no one ever mentioned to me that this was a thing.

I now understand my glycogen stores simply couldn't carry me though a full night because my body was burning them all up within a few hours no matter what I ate.

Excessive Exercise

As I've already mentioned, your metabolic processes (the ways your body uses the energy in the foods you eat) in recovery from AN are considerably different from those of a healthy person.

In recovery from AN, a disproportionate amount of energy is channelled into metabolism but also into heat generation and digestion.

To put this into context, a healthy person typically expends about ten percent of total energy (TEE) on all the processes involved with food digestion. In comparison, the energy someone in recovery from AN expends on the same digestive processes can increase three-fold or account for up to thirty percent of TEE.

In a healthy person, the remaining ninety percent of TEE (minus the ten percent used in digesting food) is split between physical activity and basal metabolic rate (BMR).

BMR is the amount of energy your body needs to carry out all its processes to survive, such as brain function, keeping your heart beating, and your lungs exchanging oxygen and carbon dioxide.

In comparison, someone recovering from AN, who is eating the same amount of energy (kilojoules/calories), will only have seventy percent of that available energy to go toward physical activity and BMR (because thirty percent of their TEE is taken up by digestion) and given that BMR is also highly elevated (due to hypermetabolism), you can see that their body is working hard.

This means there is very little (if any) spare energy for physical activity, let alone exercise.

If you are in recovery from AN, your energy needs are already greatly elevated, your heart and all your organs are severely compromised, and they are already working at full capacity. To consider exercise on top of this can triple the amount of calories necessary for weight maintenance, let alone weight gain or repair of physical damage.

If you are exercising in a malnourished or underweight state, it's not healthy. Your body is suffering.

If you are exercising in a malnourished or underweight state, damage is occurring rapidly every time you exercise, and while your body is amazing with what it can endure and repair, it does have a limit. Irreversible damage is only a matter of time.

Would you want your sister, brother, friend, mother, or father to be exercising as you are if they were sick, or would you want them to take the time out to heal?

Healthy people take time off to heal, and they don't question it. Healthy people tell others they need to rest, and they make certain that they take the best care of themselves, irrespective of what anyone else is doing.

On top of the physical dangers of exercising in a malnourished state, there is the problem that continuing to follow those compulsions perpetuates the exercise obsession.

Addiction

A useful way to think about the treatment for exercise addiction is in the same way you would treat a drug or alcohol addiction.

We don't tell alcoholics or drug addicts to try having a little bit of alcohol/drug but just don't feel addicted, do we?

"Just do it but don't let it be an addiction" is not useful advice because we know logically this isn't possible, and any amount of alcohol or drug is going to fuel the addiction. That is until that addiction has been overcome.

It is the same with exercise. You can't continue to exercise and just not feel compelled to do it because you don't want to feel compelled to do it. It's not mind over matter. Addictions, compulsions, and habits are not intellectual.

Exercise and starvation have been shown in the brains of both animals and humans to create a very similar effect to the reward system of drug addiction, including release of beta-endorphins and dopamine[62,63]. Therefore, from a most fundamental level, stopping exercise is not going to feel good.

The truth is when you are as sick as you are with AN, it doesn't matter how much you enjoy exercise if you are doing it excessively at an unhealthy weight or undereating for the amount of exercise you are doing. It is the illness ruling you, and until you recover completely, exercise is not healthy.

Your body is exhausted, and an otherwise healthy person who is malnourished due to the consequences of an illness such as cancer wouldn't be pushing themselves to exercise. I know for you it's not pushing, it's a compulsion and actually the opposite in that it is an effort to not exercise, but it is something you must face and change if you truly want your life back.

Stopping exercise was the hardest decision I have ever made.

Which is a very strange thing to say given all the hard decisions I've made in my life. I can't connect to it being the hardest at this point in time but I know for the past Bonnie who made the decision and followed though with it it was.

The reality is if the thought of stopping exercising for a period causes you distress or panic, then this is the best indication you could ask for to let you know that you really do need to stop, because it shouldn't be so emotional.

Not just stop and you're all better but stop and take time to develop a healthy relationship with yourself in which you can easily read and respond to your body's needs.

Stop and redevelop a connection to yourself that allows you to later in your life be entirely free to move your body in a way that genuinely feels good to you.

Digestive Problems

Fact: During recovery, you will experience digestive problems.

If there was one thing I could help people in recovery understand more than anything else, it would be this: that no matter how gentle you are, no matter how slow you take it, no matter what foods you eat, when, where, how, and why you eat, you will be uncomfortable.

While there is much we can do to lessen this, the reality is it can't be completely removed.

When you start increasing your food intake, all sorts of GI problems will manifest themselves. Many of them the result of the pure emotional distress and turmoil that comes with each mouthful of food, because stressful thoughts literally change the function of every system in your body and perhaps none more so than the process of digestion.

Stress activates the sympathetic nervous system, which is responsible for the release of the stress hormones and creates what you might have heard referred to as the freeze, fight, or flight response. The activation of the sympathetic nervous system shuts off the parasympathetic nervous system, the part of the nervous system which is responsible for resting and digesting.

It is well known that this stress response is an ancient adaptation to mobilise energy and divert it to where it's needed (skeletal muscles), allowing you to respond with either freezing, running, or fighting anything which is a threat to your life.

The logic being that it's not of importance that you waste energy on digesting what's in your GI tract if a sabre tooth tiger is chasing you. It is of far more importance that your muscles have the energy to run.

The freeze, fight or flight response is not within our conscious control, which is why you can't just tell yourself to relax and eat when your body is automatically running a stress response to food.

Persistent stress causes all sorts of GI problems. Slow digestion being one that is acutely uncomfortable for people with AN because their gut-brain axis is often hyper-sensitive, meaning any distention of the stomach or intestines sets off extreme anxiety, and for this to be prolonged is cruel.

Cruel but inevitable.

Ask yourself, if you knew that eating regularly and adequately would be the only way to fully rectify this hypersensitivity and to one day truly not be concerned over what you felt in your stomach before, during, or after eating, would you do it?

Because it's true.

On top of the digestive problems associated with stress, other problems occur, because your GI tract is out of practice, because the muscles of your GI tract have atrophied (been broken down) due to underuse and your body has repurposed the proteins from the smooth muscle for the more vital functions we discussed earlier.

What this all means is that during nutritional replenishment, you will likely experience uncomfortably fullness and bloating. You might feel nauseous every time you are faced with food or in pain after you eat, your oesophagus may spasm and you might have severe diarrhoea or alternate between constipation and diarrhoea.

All these symptoms will pass, but they will only pass if you persevere with renourishment. If you back down and avoid eating or restrict your food intake, you may supress the symptoms and alleviate pain in the moment, but you are not treating the cause.

Ultimately, by choosing the fleeting reprieve of restriction, you are prolonging your time to recovery, and any prolonging of your time to recovery is putting your life on hold.

Elimination Diets are Contraindicated in People with a History of an ED

Digestive complications and problems such as irritable bowel syndrome (IBS) can develop due to restrictive eating and even continue to persist after recovery.

I know the feeling of just wanting to find the answer to the physical pain. I know the feeling of just wanting to find the thing to cut out that would make it all better. However, what I know now is it's the opposite. Elimination diets are contraindicated in people with a history of an ED.

Which means, don't do it.

Please do not try to control your digestive problems through eliminating or altering your food intake (unless you are working closely with an ED dietitian).

We know with certainty that IBS is not all about the food you're eating or not eating, and there are plenty of other ways to lessen IBS symptoms other than through manipulating your food intake. If you are living with or in recovery from an ED it is highly unlikely that your IBS symptoms are solely manifesting due to an intolerance and far more likely that they are the bi-product of prolonged stress.

There is an extensive list of things that have been shown to lessen IBS symptoms outside of changing what you eat. Many of them also dealing with the root cause rather than temporary relief which you may like to consider. The include clinical hypnotherapy, neurolinguistic programming (NLP), CBT, mindfulness, meditation, yoga, medications, giving yourself time to eat meals, probiotics, massage, hot water bottles, loose clothing, getting good sleep and adequate rest, as well as gentle movement.

The blaringly obvious one though is getting through recovery. When you recover and are taking care of yourself, eating naturally, easily, and effortlessly, you will find many of the symptoms clear up on their own or simply won't be all-consuming any longer.

Therefore, while you're in recovery, certainly give techniques or medications a go and find which ones work best for you to lessen the uncomfortable symptoms, but also keep in mind that there is no way to make eating during recovery truly comfortable (and if it is, then you're probably not eating enough).

Exhaustion & Irritability

In the depths of AN, I found I had excessive energy. My body was in fight or flight mode twenty-four/seven, even I suspect when I slept, because my sleeping was so different to what it is now.

In a way, I feel like I didn't really and truly sleep for those fifteen years, because my body never fully relaxed. I literally felt ready to run at any second every second of the day. My whole body was tight and taught and ready to flee or fight.

I was relentlessly trying to do everything and please everyone, and I couldn't allow myself to feel tired.

I've read studies that indicate people with AN have vastly increased pain thresholds, which means they just don't feel pain where others would; and through my own experience, this explains a lot.

I could take guesses as to why this may be the case and I would have to include in there a component of it is most likely due to having an underdeveloped sense of self and parts of the brain associated with self-awareness, which would create a lack of ability to perceive inputs associated with self, including pain. Which means it's not only that you ignore pain but also that a pain stimulus is perceived as less painful to you than the same stimulus would be perceived in a healthy person.

In part, I would also trace this increased pain threshold to the natural stress response I spoke about earlier in terms of fight or flight. We know when stressed and faced with a life-or-death situation, animals, including humans, are able to withstand great pain they wouldn't otherwise be able to because of the release of hormones such as adrenaline.

Living with AN or in recovery from AN is a prolonged stress response.

Would you be willing to consider letting go of the increased pain threshold superpower thing and panicky excessive energy thing if it meant you got a chance at a real and authentic life?

This is something I legitimately asked myself, because they were both things I prided myself on long before I knew they were linked to AN. My ability to endure without complaint was something I was secretly and misguidedly proud of.

Consider asking yourself the same question now.

At some stage, as you develop your sense of self, you learn to recognise what you are feeling, and when you do so, you will realise you're tired.

Exhausted, in fact.

There's no possible way to not be, with what your body, mind, and soul have been through and are going through.

At some stage, you will have to learn to respond to this in a healthful way, because the big picture goal of recovery is to become a "healthy" person.

You must get the help you need to let go of the relentless pushing, pushing, pushing (including when, to you, the pushing feels normal) and learn to recognise and respond to your body.

I found there came a point when recovery itself hit me. I realised I was exhausted. It felt like the ways I had abused my body (for the most part unintentionally) caught up with me all in one go. Mentally and physically, I hit a wall. I was suddenly unable to push myself the way I had for years.

I felt confused, ashamed, frustrated, and mad at myself for my sudden lack of energy. I felt lazy and disgusted that my body and mind were suddenly so weak, as I saw it.

This alone made me run back to the AN behaviours more than once because it reinforced to me that without anorexia, I would be lazy, unmotivated, achieve nothing, be an utterly useless and pathetic waste of space with no drive and amount to nothing. It reinforced that AN was a good thing about me.

All these fears were eventually exposed for what they were; pure nonsense or in kinder terms "non-useful beliefs". They were the noise of a scared and confused mind.

Micronutrient Deficiencies

Throughout recovery, you must get regular blood tests to monitor your BGLs, nutrient levels, and electrolytes (such as sodium and potassium).

A study published in 2017 concluded with strong support in favour for the collection of a routine full blood count, electrolytes, phosphate, liver function tests, cholesterol, vitamin B12, red cell folate, vitamin D, magnesium, zinc, and manganese at initial presentation[63].

However, even if your blood work always comes back within the "normal" range, it actually does not mean you are fine.

Your blood is what connects every part of your body, and your body works very hard to keep it all looking good. Which means that just because your blood contains nutrients within the healthy range does not mean that your cells are getting access to or utilising those substances.

Correcting Nutritional Deficiencies

Some of your nutritional deficiencies, if they have been prolonged, may have reached the point where you won't be able to rectify them through dietary improvements alone.

I will just give one example of what I mean here. A deficiency in vitamin B12 which can cause macrocytic anaemia, lethargy, irritability, weakness, and if left untreated can lead to paralysis, irreversible brain damage, and even death, will unlikely be achievable through food alone.

Severe B12 deficiency requires at least a course of three B12 injections to get your levels back up within a healthy range. After which you will only then be able to go on to meet your needs and maintain your levels through adequate food intake.

Don't Overcomplicate It (Don't Even Complicate It)
As your body is going through the exhaustion of weight gain and repair of physical damage, there are biological reasons for everything you are experiencing.

Which means you are just getting in your own way when you try to make it mean anything more complicated than this.

Don't make it personal, because it's not personal.

Your body is a human body, and like any other human body having gone through starvation and malnutrition, it has things it needs to do in order to heal.

Let it.

Conclusion to Stage One: Surrender - Weight Gain and Repair of Physical Damage

Change will lead to insight far more often than insight will lead to change.
~ Milton Erickson

The process of weight gain takes time. Physical repair takes longer still. Neither weight gain nor repair of physical damage can be avoided, nor can they be rushed. There are no shortcuts to healing. You certainly can put your all into it and heal much faster, but what you can't do is heal before you're healed.

There are no shortcuts to recovery because there are no shortcuts to a healthy, happy, and fulfilling life. That is a lifelong process.

It is only when you are out of starvation, out of malnutrition, and your body trusts that it is not going to be starved again that you can truly advance with the second and most exciting part of recovery; growth.

This second stage of recovery is where your mind and body will be switching back on and where you will be coming to life. This stage is your opportunity not for recovering to some former self but for growth beyond what you've ever known.

Stage Two of Recovery: Growth

Component Three - Psychological Development

When you do really stupid stuff, you have to learn to stop it and do something better.
~ Richard Bandler

Introduction to Psychological Development
While AN may manifest in your body as a physical illness, never is it purely a physical illness.

Psychological development is the stage of recovery which addresses the one factor which will change everything, your mind.

In full recovery, your mind is on board, allowing you to become fully competent, capable, and confident to care for yourself, both now and for the rest of your life, because until the care comes completely from your own psychology, it is of limited value.

Where Recovery Stops is Where Your Life Begins

No amount of action can compensate for how you really feel.
~ Bonnie Killip

Although all three components of recovery overlap, intertwine, and coincide with one another, I have left psychological development as the final stage because from a place of starvation, psychological development simply is not possible, and from a place of malnutrition and fear, it is severely limited.

In the beginning of recovery, safety, security, and certainty are your highest priorities.

Your focus is dominated by escaping the suffering, and you can't imagine a greater dream than to simply be free or to feel "normal".

As you progress, and the need for safety, security, and certainty are consistently maintained and your physical health improves, both what you want and what you are capable of expand.

When you are starving, although it is a great deal harder, you can learn, you can understand the theory, you can see the value, but what you can't do is the most important part, which is apply the knowledge, otherwise known as "do it".

It is not until you are reasonably nourished that you will be capable of the "real doing," because your brain, as a human brain, requires a decent level of nutritional replenishment to function in the ways you will be asking it to.

In this second stage of recovery (growth) and third and final component of recovery (psychological development), the focus shifts from escaping to creating. You naturally, rather than force yourself, choose exploration. When you reach this stage, you must now reset your goals, because safety and security are no longer going to cut it.

I liken this second stage of recovery to a child learning about the world, and it really is like this; seeing the world through an entirely new lens, which is why I've termed it "growth".

The sense you need to call upon most to be successful at growth is "curiosity".

Growth is about dropping the judgement and stepping into curiosity.

It is in this stage where my thoughts changed from "when will recovery be over?" to "how far can I go?" Because while right now, to not be sick may be your highest goal and dream of what is possible, but this is actually not the end, it is the beginning.

This is where your life really begins.

What Do I Do Now?

We all have two lives. The second begins when we realise, we have only one.
~ Confucius

Interestingly, even though this expansion is what you want and what you've worked so hard for, it can be just as terrifying and overwhelming as the constrictive world you lived in with AN. It's just that it is terrifying and overwhelming in other ways. It may seem unbelievable, but it's true, and to leave this unacknowledged would be leaving out a significant truth of recovery.

Living with AN means you have become accustomed to living by rules, recovery itself has rules and there is certainty in rules.

What to do now is far less clear.

You Don't Know What You Don't Know

Shame shields solutions.
~ Tiffany Aliche

It is now that I highly encourage you to have a strong support team by your side. What you need now is very different than what you needed in the early stages of recovery.

Too often, people in recovery from EDs are offered support for the first stage of recovery and then when they're ready for stage two are left to fend on their own.

What to do here, when the person is no longer considered a medical emergency and is out of obvious physical danger, is far less clear and hard to address. At least, that is, from the medical model from which AN is traditionally solely treated.

If you are feeling as though your hope in your ability to recover is being eroded, you've been here before or maybe a part of you suspects this system has offered you all it has to offer, it's not an indication of any failing on your behalf or that you're incapable of recovery. Please don't waste your time getting caught up in the just telling yourself you need to try harder. Take it as the evidence you need that you must now look outside this model.

What is Psychological Development?

Most people are f*cked up because they're doing stupid s*it inside their minds.
~ Richard Bandler

Living with AN, you may have come to fear your mind. Living with anorexia means your thoughts and your feelings are unpredictable and completely beyond your control. But what if I were to share with you that the opposite is also true and you can gain a great deal more control over what you think, feel, and therefore do then maybe you've ever experienced before?

Imagine if you had a way of trusting yourself, with complete certainty to always choose the option that would allow you to think, feel, and act in ways which were good for you, irrespective of how anyone in the outside world treated you, and at the same time feel good doing it; no guilt, no shame, and no excruciating self-doubt and judgement?

This is where psychological development will get you, because psychological development is about adding choices.

Health and Well-being for Life

Self-care is giving the world the best of you, instead of what is left of you.
~ Katie Reed

Psychological development is where you get to create the environment, both internal and external, that will support your health and well-being for life.

As you move from the surrender stage of recovery to the growth stage, you are truly embarking on nothing less than the greatest opportunity of a lifetime.

The Opportunity of a Lifetime

Beauty is in the eye of the beholder.
~ Margaret Wolfe Hungerford

During recovery, not only will you be building a new body, you are also building a new mind. This is the part where you get to intentionally free yourself to discover, create, and become more you. This is something many people never get the opportunity to do.

For most people, this happens passively (as it has for you up until this point), which means they don't get a say, to the degree they could, in who they would like to be.

We all have things "put there" by the way our mind interprets things, and the way our mind interprets things depends on our capabilities and understandings at any given time.

In the growth stage of recovery, you have the opportunity now and every moment thereafter until the day you leave this world to consciously be aware of and decide who and what you want to be.

Importantly, you get to go about living to that. You get to experience the freedom that is simply being you.

The pain you went through to achieve this will one day pale in comparison to the rich and full life you now live, this I know.

Psychological Development is the Key to Recovery

Do or do not, there is no try.
~ Yoda

To understand why psychological development is so important, I am going to share with you a little more of my story.

Once upon a time in a kingdom far, far away that wasn't very magical, I believed weight gain equalled recovery.

My recovery attempts were always highly focussed on reaching a certain weight (prescribed to me by the outside world).

I went into weight gain each and every time with positivity and high hopes, because everything and anything must be better than this starved, anxious, and fearful state I was living in.

I would commit to gaining weight with a drive and determination second to none, and the initial stages were intoxicating. There was a phenomenal freedom that came with unconditional permission to eat. It was incredible to feel the energy coursing through my veins, to feel the changes as my body and mind came to life, and the wide expanses of possibility open up before me.

However, relatively quickly, it would become increasingly difficult to continue, because while consciously I wanted to gain weight, it never felt right to do the things which helped me gain weight for any reason outside of the purpose of gaining weight.

The further I got from the impending fear of death or rehospitalisation, the less compelling weight gain became, and yet I would persevere because everything and everyone insisted it would get easier.

It didn't.

Time and time again, I pushed myself and I hurt myself until I would eventually reach that magical number. And time and time again, I would lose it all, in what truly felt like the blink of an eye.

It was almost a sense of "mission complete, what now"?

To which I had no answer, and my mind defaulted back to what it knew best. The ED.

Temporary Body

I didn't know, and I mean I had no clue, what to do when I got to this magical weight to stay there.

I wouldn't even know when I was there, because I still saw myself as thin, frail, scared, broken, and incapable.

I felt like a fraud. I felt like a fake. This "healthy" body wasn't me. Therefore, I couldn't maintain it. That body was only ever temporary. To keep it would have taken a monumental daily effort, and I didn't have that in me every day for the rest of my lifetime.

No one does.

I lacked the psychological development necessary for healthy, to feel okay, let alone come naturally or even be, God forbid, enjoyable.

Child at The Wheel

Fear makes the wolf bigger than he is.
~ African Proverb.

I was told innumerable times that once I gained weight, my brain would be better, and there is no denying that it was; my brain was stronger, but when it was stronger, it also wanted more.

It would come to a point where the wonderous effects of renourishment could get me no further, and I now had this fully nourished brain that was no kinder to me than before I'd gained the weight.

Furthermore, having lived with an ED for so long meant the life I had built wasn't necessarily authentically mine. It was a half-hearted, fear filled, foundation less life filled with things I never truly chose. Much of it felt meaningless.

I would then blame myself that I wasn't getting better, that I was beyond hope, because everyone and everything insisted this weight gain was what would make me better.

I was failing at the ED, and I was failing at recovery. It felt like there was no place for me.

Really, I was just a child behind the control panel of the most powerful machine in the universe, and there was a very limited number of things I knew how to do. My treatment never updated along with where I was mentally.

It is only now, looking back, that I can see that this was because no one I ever sought help from knew how to help with this stage. I was always treated as a chronically ill patient. I was always treated as someone with an illness that was impossible to recover from. I was always treated as though the only reason I wasn't recovering was because I didn't want to recover. Clearly a conflicting, confusing, and arguably impossible place to recover from.

Neuroplasticity and Neural Rewiring

> *The way to get started is to quit talking and begin doing.*
> *~ Walt Disney*

In hindsight I can see I was taking advice from well-meaning but equally lost people. Advice which was necessary in the first two components of recovery (weight gain and repair of physical damage) but which was no longer helpful because as my brain switched back on, my needs were now vastly different.

The behaviours of anorexia were so ingrained and so much a part of me that the very neurology of my brain needed to be changed, and that, unfortunately, does not change spontaneously through refeeding alone.

I needed guidance on how to learn to take effective and healthy leadership of my life. Not from an intellectual level, because I'd read the books, I'd talked about it, I'd reasoned it out with myself, and I'd even done the university degrees that gave me the credentials to help others in my position. The intellectual understanding was not the problem. What I needed was help to change at a neurological level. I needed help to develop my capable self-identity, my sense of self-worth and belonging in the world, because without this, any weight gain, any "health" gain, could only ever be fleeting.

Gaining knowledge and learning is not so difficult. For the most part, it's quite enjoyable because it gives us a sense that we're doing something productive and important. Crucially, it is also safe. However, it is the transition from knowledge to action where all the real power of recovery lives, and that was where I just couldn't find anyone who could help.

And I wasn't much help to myself because I knew a lot but I didn't know what I didn't know…

If you're experiencing similar challenges, perhaps psychological development is the step you're most ready for, because if you gain weight and develop the knowledge and the skills, you will go forward. If you gain weight and don't develop the knowledge and skills, you will retreat.

This is not a choice, it is biological.

Welcome to Real

Do not think of yourself as the body but as the joyous consciousness and the immortal behind it.
~ Paramahansa Yogananda

If you feel stuck in the perpetual cycle of weight gain and loss, feel something is missing, that you are dependent on others for your health, or feel that if left alone you doubt you would be capable of caring for yourself, this is okay. There is no need to fight against where you are or pretend it is any other way, but far from meaning you are broken or that this is permanent, it actually means it is the psychological development part which you are now ready for.

Your recovery need not be all about fear, scarcity, and uncertainty any longer.

Welcome to the fun part. Also, the hard part but without question the part that makes it all "worth it". The part that anyone who has ever lived with an eating disorder is most interested in.

Prelude to the 6 Areas of Psychological Development

The best and most beautiful things in the world cannot be seen or even touched – they must be felt with the heart.
~ Helen Keller

Before I introduce the 6 areas of psychological development and dive into explanations of each and how you can begin to build them into your recovery and your life going forward from today, I want to share an analogy with you.

I share this analogy as a means of introducing and clarifying a few of the concepts I will be talking about in this section, including beliefs, capabilities, and self-identity, because these concepts can be hard to understand if you haven't had much to do with them before. I know the first time I was introduced to them as things that were changeable, it certainly was difficult for me to understand.

A Magical Analogy

You can create beyond what has been and what is, only by imagining beyond what has been and what is.
~ Bonnie Killip

One of the most foundational changes of psychological development has to do with changing your limiting beliefs to empowering beliefs. This can be thought of a little like the beginning of the Harry Potter series (if you haven't read or seen them, that's okay, you'll be able to follow along. If you haven't read them but intend to this is a spoiler alert).

Harry Potter is the story of a boy who grows up being abused by his aunt, uncle, and cousin after his own parents are murdered when he is a baby. At the age of eleven, Harry is told by a stranger that he is a wizard, and not only a wizard but a wizard who is famous in the magical world.

At the time when Harry receives his letter of offer to attend Hogwarts School of Witchcraft and Wizardry, he has no idea he is a wizard. He, therefore, has no comprehension of the powers he has within him.

Even when he has a letter inviting him to study at the school in his own hands (proof), he does not believe it, because his beliefs (what he holds to be true), which he has learned passively through his environment (living with his abusive aunt, uncle, and cousin) up until that point have been that he has very low value. In fact, his level of disbelief in an alternate reality is in such a high level of contradiction with his current map of reality that he thinks there is a mistake.

Essentially, Harry has limiting beliefs and a low sense of self, which, however true they are in his mind, do not match the reality of the depth of his powers.

If your recovery is anything like mine (or Harry's coming to realise he is a wizard), you will start in a place of having an exceptionally low sense of self, including a low sense of self-worth, self-esteem, self-confidence, self-belief, self-trust and almost non-existent self-capabilities (even if logically you know this is not true, part of you tells you it is true).

I'll just emphasise that you don't have to grow up being abused to develop these beliefs there are many other ways we come to such conclusions (for example maybe low self-worth was modelled to us by a parent who was always putting themselves or even others down).

You are unlikely to think of yourself as anything special (certainly not magical), and maybe you even think AN gives you something special and without it you would have and be nothing remarkable at all.

Then, as you start down the road of recovery and find a treatment team who believe in you and treat you as though you are capable and their conviction in your capabilities and beliefs is unshakable, your mind will begin to increasingly question and release the limiting beliefs of AN.

Eventually, Harry does come to understand and believe he has powers and that he is capable, thanks in part to Hagrid's (your treatment team, whether that is one person or ten people) conviction and strong belief in him (you).

However, this is far from where the story ends, because while Harry may now believe he has these powers, he still needs to go to school to learn how to use them effectively.

Similarly, when you believe you are strong, powerful, and capable (through nutritional support and doing the work to change your limiting beliefs to capable and empowering beliefs. Which is work beyond people just telling you you are or treating you as though you are), you will move on to the need for guidance on how to develop and grow your powers.

Now, you can head off to wizard school (where you get to utilise professional guidance on psychological development) to learn how to use all the magic that is already within you and to learn new magic you don't yet know.

Imagine learning you had magical powers and heading off to magic school. Take a moment to imagine this fully and completely. Imagine learning you were someone else all along. Imagine learning that differentness you felt within you was because you were magical.

On top of learning how to use your magic, it is time now to update or create a new self-identity, because just as Harry's old self-identity as the orphan living in the cupboard under the stairs at the house of people who despised him, with nothing remarkable about him had to change for him to function in the wizard world, so does the way you perceive yourself.

You're no longer that person. How does it feel to know that? Exciting? Terrifying? A bit of both (plus some)?

Honestly, the loss of identity is one of the most terrifying parts of recovery, but this is a position you will find yourself faced with if full recovery is your goal.

The creation or the update of a new self-identity and not just the loss of an old identity is necessary.

There are times when it will be tough.

Remember, at times even Harry, Ron, and Hermine (Harry's two best friends he meets at wizard school) complain about learning magic (I truly never understood their complaints about homework that involved learning MAGIC!), but overall, learning how to use your powers is fun and unquestionably rewarding.

When you believe in your capabilities, you next need to practice them. As you practice new ways of being in the world, you prove to yourself that your beliefs are true (or at least a more useful truth) and vice versa, because your new capabilities will form new beliefs, and your new capabilities are endless… Life is not done when you recover from an eating disorder.

This is the continuation of psychological development into your life for the rest of your life. You will never stop advancing, and there'll always be little challenges or big challenges (Voldemort who is the evil character in the Harry Potter series certainly hung around for a long time, didn't he?), but the important thing is you are now aware of your magic, and you are intentionally growing and supporting you.

There you have it, a brief magical analogy to introduce some of the key concepts of psychological development, which I am now dedicating the next few pages to explaining in further depth.

3.3 Introducing the 6 Areas of Psychological Development

What you get by achieving your goals is not as important as what you become by achieving your goals.
~ Zig Ziglar

In the interest of simplifying and clarifying what can feel like a monumental talk there are six areas I see as essential to successful psychological development (otherwise known as transformation). Similar to the Two-Stage Model of Recovery the first three are primarily associated with building and breaking-free, and the second three are generative and focused on growth and expansion.

Breaking-free

- Welcome It
- Decide
- Get Clear on What You Want

Growth

- Creating Empowering Beliefs
- Developing your Capable Self-Identity
- Giving yourself Unconditional Permission

1. Welcome It

You cannot fix a problem you are not first willing to have.

~ Bonnie Killip

When I first wrote this book, this first step of psychological development was titled very differently. It was titled "Separate Yourself from the ED". I cringe a little at the thought, but I also believe it's important to share with you because it is the most common way of thinking when it comes to ED recovery, and consequently one of the most common ways that EDs are treated. It was one of the things I had been told to do, time and time again throughout my recovery.

When I was thirteen, a psychologist wrote "It" on a piece of paper and told me to take that paper and put it somewhere else when the ED thoughts came up. I had no clue what she meant, because at that time I didn't see a separation. The ED was me.

Even if I could have been capable of making a distinction, there was no way I'd have been able to separate "It" from me and not have those feelings simply by putting a piece of paper away from me.

From a perspective of limited understanding, it does make sense why a model of treatment which encourages people to separate themselves from the ED would be used. However, re-reading this section (more than a year after I first wrote it), it hit me that this type of thinking had been less than useful to me, and in the end, it was the opposite which healed me.

So, I've decided rather than perpetuate that mostly outdated model, I'm going to share with you what helped me.

What I came to learn through my recovery and my life since recovered is that the ED, despite very much appearing so, was never there to ruin my life or sabotage my efforts. In fact, it existed for the very opposite.

It was trying to help me.

Anorexia Nervosa is Not a Monster

Your conflicts, all the difficult things, the problematic situations in your life, are not chance or haphazard. They are actually yours. They are specifically yours, designed specifically for you by a part of you that loves you more than anything else.
The part of you that loves you more than anything else has created roadblocks to lead you to yourself.
You are not going in the right direction unless there is something pricking you in the side, telling you, "Look here! This way!" That part of you loves you so much that it doesn't want you to lose the chance. It will go to extreme measures to wake you up, it will make you suffer greatly if you don't listen.
What else can it do? That is its purpose.
~ A. H Almaas

You did not create AN in your life. The ED and all the thoughts and behaviours that follow are often initially formed in response to an emotional learning.

In other words, it is a way your brain created to make sense of and cope with a specific set of circumstances or experiences at a time in your past when you had no other way of coping.

You got sick in response to life events big or small, seemingly insignificant or monumental, it does not matter, because your mind developed this way of protecting you from things you had no other way of dealing with at that time.

When viewed in this light, the ED is not a pathology, a malfunction, the enemy, or a monster but a way in which your brain evolved to survive in this world the best way it knew how.

You can hate what the ED has done, but know that at the core, its intentions were always and still are what that part of you thought and thinks are best for you. It has at its core the very best of intentions for you. Because it is you.

The problem is your mind hasn't updated to the situation you're now in. Your brain hasn't fully got that the ED way of doing things isn't truly successful at achieving what it wanted to achieve through doing it in the first place. Your mind hasn't fully got that those ways of thinking, feeling, and behaving are no longer necessary because you're now capable of more useful ways.

Which means it is preferred if you update your mind in light of the new information and experiences you've had in your rich life. Because by allowing your thoughts, feelings, and actions to be dictated by your past won't give you the present nor the future you're capable of.

Rather than destroying or fighting against it, give welcoming this hurt and scared part of you a shot. Let this part know it's okay to speak up. Thank it for all it has done and allow it to enter the conversation.

You must stop running.

You must stop ignoring.

You must stop avoiding.

You must stop hiding.

You must stop downplaying.

You must stop putting off and, you must now…

2. Decide

The cycle won't stop, you must get off.
~ Bonnie Killip

Honesty

You are not going to reach a stage where the ED tells you "Okay, you are sick enough, you can go and get help and recover now".

The ED isn't going anywhere until you choose to face it and decide to change.

To change you must first accept exactly where you are in this moment, regardless of where you've been or where you want to be, and this requires being completely honest with yourself.

Acceptance is not Resignation

> *Once we accept our limits, we go beyond them.*
>
> *~ Albert Einstein*

If you have been trying to recover for years, consider trying something different. Consider trying something revolutionary and stop trying to be beyond where you are.

Accepting where you are does not mean that you create comfort in where you are, nor that you are declaring defeat and resigning yourself to staying there forever. What is does mean is that you give yourself permission to be exactly where you are, exactly as you. It is this compassionate acceptance which allows you to give your body adequate time to rest and heal and finally begin to move out of where you are, because the problem you may find is not so much where you are as it is your judgement of where you are (a failure, not good enough, embarrassed, ashamed, guilty, regretful).

Now is your time to drop the judgement.

Imagine how much simpler it would all be if you did not feel that confusing mix of emotions. Imagine if you recognised you had a problem and went about using your energy to learn and practice ways to move forward.

Admit You Don't Know How

> *Surrender your fear, something will come that is far greater than what the fear is trying to protect.*
>
> *~ Moojr*

I made the decision to stop trying to convince, reassure, and protect others by insisting I was capable and that I was doing the right thing and instead owned the fact that I wasn't and that I didn't know how to most of the time. But I was willing to learn and most importantly I was willing to learn imperfectly.

I was an adult when I recovered from AN, but I was a child in many ways. I had missed almost fifteen crucial years of learning how to be an adult. My entire adult life had been taken up by the illness.

I had little concept of what life on the other side of sickness would be, even as I wanted it and strived after it.

The sheer volume of things I thought I had to learn in order to be recovered and survive in this world was overwhelming. The overwhelm kept me paralysed.

Those things I pressured myself into needing to know "now" were not all overdramatic, and many of them were true and realistic things I did need to learn but I couldn't have ever learned them by staying in the illness and trying to learn them and only moving forward once I had. I could only have learned them the way I did (and still am); through doing them (stuffing up, succeeding, stuffing up, and trying again).

Busy, Busy, Busy

Everybody thinks of changing the world, but no one thinks of changing himself.
~ Leo Tolstoy

When I was sick and striving for recovery, I hoped that if I kept busy enough, if I filled my life with numerous other things, I would eventually leave no space for AN. I thought I could do more and more and more until it would be squeezed out of existence.

To put it bluntly, it is ignorant and at the very least immature to think you can do away with AN purely at the behavioural level.

The reality is you are far more complicated than that, and the ED isn't going anywhere until you have other choices in how to think, feel, and behave. No matter how many other things you fill your life with.

Validation is Not Where Your Healing Is

Patients enter therapy, not to cure their neuroses, but to perfect them.
~ Karen Horney

Deciding to recover is about knowing you have valid reasons for doing what you're doing and choosing to release them anyway.

Think about it this way: Would you rather the world understands and accommodates to things you don't even want to be thinking, feeling, or doing because you have legitimate reasons for thinking, feeling and doing them, or would you rather learn how to stop doing them (and insread do what you do want to be doing)?

Do not waste your time and energy on insisting others validate your illness. Even if you were to get all the validation in the world, validation is not where your healing is.

Recovery is About Creating a Life You do Not Need Distraction From

No amount of self-improvement can make up for a lack of self-acceptance.
~ Robert Holden

During my time in "recovery", I attempted numerous forms of "treatment", and many of them promoted techniques of distraction, avoidance, and "stress relief".

Looking back now, it is a huge shame to me that this was what I was taught, because while these are all valuable and have a place, they are only tools for temporary relief.

What I needed was to face the stress, recognise what I was stressed about, and learn the skills to deal with the stress, not just ignore, distract, or block it out for a time.

A lot of my stress was for genuine and reasonable reasons. We all have legitimate reasons for stress. No one, not a single soul, lives a stress-free existence, and no amount of distraction or stress relief can compensate for a lack of actual ability to deal with stress or, more importantly, to learn to do the things you don't know how to do that are causing you stress because you don't know how to do them.

Recovery is about creating a life you do not need distraction from. Recovery is about building the resilience to live through stress and it's about not adding unnecessary stress on top of the unavoidable stresses of life (being underfed, overexercised, and shaming yourself, to name a few ways of not even giving yourself a chance).

If You are Doing Recovery, it is Time to Do Recovery

The result is only as good as the desire and bloody enthusiasm to get it.
~ Dein Horn

If you have decided recovered is something you would like and you consider yourself in recovery, this means it is time to do recovery.

Now.

Doing recovery means no more palming it off with thoughts like "it's not that bad" or "I'm not as sick as them". Doing recovery means no more putting off the hard things until tomorrow, next week, month, or year. Doing recovery means no more "I'll change when he/she/they/society changes". Doing recovery means you have to take the conditions off of when you will recover, because without pretence and without hiding, this is your life now.

Your recovery is your responsibility. Decide to do it or decide to not do it, but don't stay forever in indecision, because by not making a decision, you are making a decision.

3. **Know What You Want (Discovering and Living to Your Values)**

Run toward happiness, not just away from pain.

~ Bonnie Killip

Imagine for a moment that you have welcomed AN, you have made the decision to recover, and you are now facing it all without running, without pretending, protecting, or hiding. What now?

What do you want when your purpose is no longer fighting the illness? What will your life look like when you're no longer planning it around the limitations of AN? What are you going to be thinking, feeling, and doing when you're no longer running from pain?

You're not going to have any of the AN thoughts or behaviours when you are recovered, which means you must decide what you do want in the space they took up, and that's a whole lot of space.

Now is your time to discover.

Creating a Compelling Future

Tragedy is a tool for the living to gain wisdom, not a guide by which to live.
~ Robert Kennedy

By learning what you want, you take the first steps in creating a meaningful and fulfilling life outside of the ED. A life into which you are drawn. A life into which you are compelled and excited to get into experiencing.

After all, the point of recovery is not to recover into the very same life which created or perpetuated the illness in the first place.

It is to create and live a life that is good enough for you. Not perfect but good enough.

Forward Focused

Fighting illness does not create health, creating health creates health.
~ Bonnie Killip

Knowing what you want is much more useful than knowing about the illness. You can become an expert on AN, but if you're an expert on AN and only learning about AN, that doesn't leave much room for the new (the important part), does it?

You know how to do AN. You've done it very well for, if you're reading this book, likely years. You've got all the information you need on how to do that. What you need now is the information and practice on being healthy.

In order to meet your needs and recover, you must stop fighting illness and instead focus your energy on learning and building what you need, because the fact that the ED persists means there are some skills or resources you've yet to develop.

Think of it like a GPS; you can have the best GPS system in the world but if you only ever ask it questions about where you are or where you've been, you won't ever get information on how to get anywhere new.

You Don't Need to Be a Warrior to Be Strong or Special

You can get humans serious about just about anything, it's getting them to have fun that's the hard part.
~ Richard Bandler

Recovery is a fight, oh gosh it is, but if you are always focussed on what you must do in order to beat the pain, this detracts from the real motivator. And the real motivator is a life that is so much more than the absence of pain.

The real motivator is an authentic and fulfilling life.

What You Want, What You Really, Really Want

You might want a great job, to own your own business, to travel, a loving relationship, fulfilling work, children, more friends, to play on a sporting team, a nice car, house, or a puppy.

Whatever things you want, you must know why you want them, and the reason you want them is because having them means something to you. You might want them because you believe they will make you feel loved, appreciated, successful, happy, content, connected, significant, free, or any number of other feelings.

Therefore, knowing what you want is more so about knowing what you want to feel in your life, because everything we do and everything we want is because of a feeling. Either a feeling we want more of or a feeling we want less of.

You may have all those things and more and be lacking the feeling you want. The feelings are what you really want, the feelings let you know what you value.

Living to Your Values

Great acts are made up of small deeds.
~ Lao Tzu

If you are unsure of your values, you can't choose the option that is right for you, even if you want to. Therefore, it's time to get clear on your top values. You can then use your top values as overarching guiding principles for all decisions you make and all that you do.

Eliciting Your Values

Life is really simple, but we insist on making it complicated.
~ Confucius

If you haven't done any value work, I highly recommend you do. In fact, for recovery and for a fulfilling life, understanding your values is not only a recommendation but also a requirement.

This doesn't mean your values will never change, but do the work now, and you will live the rewards for the rest of your life.

As an introduction to values is I suggest you sit down and write a list of all the things in life that are important to you. Next, put numbers beside them in order of their importance to you. Not in order of importance in how you have lived or how you are living now but how you want to live, in a way that if you were to do so would allow you to feel the best you could feel.

Some examples of values to get you started are things like family, love, happiness, work, friendship, and money. Get specific and use as much detail as you can.

Essentially, values are those things which are important to you, with the keyword being YOU, because you won't feel fulfilled or satisfied in life until you are living in congruence with your values (not the things society, your parents, teachers, or friends have told you to value but rather those things you truly value).

For example, if you think friends are incredibly important to you, more than any of the other values on your list, and you don't currently have particularly amazing friends, go ahead and put friendship as number one.

The next step is the important part. After you've made the list, you must start going about filling your life with these things that you've identified as important to you.

You must live you life as if those things you say are important to you are indeed important to you.

If you are to live the best life you can live, you must begin to build your life around the things that you value, because when you think and act in ways that are congruent with your values, you will feel fulfilled.

Overall, remember this is a lifelong process which will shift and change as your circumstances and experiences shift and change.

Valued Traits

Another exercise which is a fun way of eliciting what you value is, is to identify those traits you value in other people. To do this, write a list of people you admire (you don't have to know them personally), then, next to their names write what it is about each of them you admire (you don't have to love everything about them).

You may be surprised by what you discover.

I know when I did this for the first time, all the people in my life that I respected and trusted were all people who it was evident knew their worth. They were all people who weren't afraid to speak up and say what they needed and wanted. I discovered I respected the strong and powerful traits most. The traits I thought were bad in myself and which I squashed down and actively suppressed were the traits I most respected in others.

Wow.

I am curious to know what you will find and even more importantly how you will use your discoveries...

The Power is in the Doing (Always)

You cannot get what you want if your only focus is on what others want for you.
~ Bonnie Killip

That is a small introduction to the theory behind values, but like everything in recovery, the theory is not where the power is. The very best way you can discover what you value, enjoy, and don't enjoy if you're not yet sure is to get out there and experiment, and when you find them, know that only you can give yourself permission to live by them.

Which brings us to the next area of psychological development; that of creating empowering beliefs.

4. Creating Empowering Beliefs

The day you believe this is a war you can win is the day you have won.
~ Bonnie Killip

Any form of coaching, if it is to be successful, begins by addressing psychology, and this is no different in recovery.

No one goes into recovery believing wholeheartedly that it's possible (or if they do believe it's possible for others, there is a list of reasons why it's not possible for them). It is along the way as you are taking steps, applying strategies, processes, or tools for health that you start to increasingly solidify the belief that change is possible.

If you believe that the new behaviours you learn will indeed get you closer to the outcome you want you're far more likely to do them. If you don't believe in the importance of your actions in getting you where you want to be, it will be harder to do them, especially when things get tough, and in recovery, things will get tough. Often.

In recovery, things *are* tough.

Another way of looking at this is, when you believe you can't do something, you might give it a try and "see what happens", but trying is not doing.

Imagine the difference between doing something because you knew it was going to lead to your recovery versus doing something you thought was pointless but you would give it a go anyway.

Notice how your feelings toward each differ. Notice the level of energy that comes with the thought of each of those options.

What we believe is foundational to our success, or not. That is why working with your beliefs in recovery is necessary. It's not the place we start but it is a place that is worth working on changing.

What Controls Your Actions?

Ask yourself, is this possible?
~ Bonnie Killip

It is what we believe about ourselves and the world more than anything else which guides our feelings, actions, capabilities, and experience of life.

Imagine if you felt differently about yourself, about the world you live in than you currently feel, do you imagine your actions would naturally change? This is essentially what recovery and sustainable health for anyone comes down to.

You can't keep the same AN thoughts and be recovered from AN. AN is a psychological illness with physical symptoms.

Think about it like this; you don't do an AN behaviour just for the sake of doing the behaviour, do you? There are strong emotions driving you to do it. There are strong emotions stopping you from not doing it. If you don't think so, then think about not doing it next time you feel you "have to" and notice what you feel in your body. Panic? Anxiety? Fear? Stress?

When we change the feelings, our behaviours automatically change, and the single most powerful way to change any feeling is through changing beliefs.

This is vastly different to positive thinking or blind optimism, because there are hard and fast ways to change beliefs. Changing and updating beliefs is a natural part of life, which means your brain naturally has the ability to do it. In recovery you are just helping it out.

Do you remember believing in Santa Clause or the Easter Bunny or something else you believed in as a child? I'm guessing if you do remember believing somewhere back there in your past, you no longer do today.

So, consider, in the same way you no longer hold those old beliefs, that even if you believe something today, for example, that you have to "earn your food" or that you are not "worthy" or "good enough", that it's possible you can no longer believe this in the future and even believe something more functional in its place, for example, that you are loved, loveable, worthy, enough...

Change Your Mind, Change Your Life

Whether you think you can or you think you can't,
you are right.
~ Henry Ford

I am one hundred percent certain that you would much rather change the way you think and feel so that you naturally change how you behave rather than continue to force yourself to change what you are doing and still feel the same pain. This concept is what this book and my entire model for recovery is based on. That recovery is about changing the underlying thought processes and beliefs which are preventing change.

It is also about creating in their place new, more empowering and useful ways of thinking and feeling, because this will allow you to have new ways of being.

The Scenario

If you could eat each meal (the behaviour) but still feel completely horrible doing it (the emotion) for the rest of your life, how likely are you to be excited and inspired by that life? How likely are you to do everything it takes to reach that life?

On the other hand, if you could change the way you feel about eating so that it was no longer painful (and even, revolutionary new territory here, enjoyable instead) how readily do you then think the behaviour to do it would follow?

Now, the question is what would you do to reach that second version of your future?

Two Kinds of Beliefs

Reality is nothing but the free choice of many doors that are open at all times.
~ P. Watawick

When I was sick, there were moments where I'd have been happy with a brain transplant or a lobotomy if either had been offered.

I drove myself crazy with all the theoretical knowledge I had of what I should be doing and yet could not get myself to apply it. Why couldn't I translate all I knew to be good for me into actions?

One of the reasons is that there are two types of beliefs.

The first type of beliefs are those we are consciously aware of. These are the beliefs we know we have.

The second type of beliefs are those we are not consciously aware of (unconscious beliefs). These are the beliefs we do not know we have.

It is the later which run our lives.

When we find ourselves stuck in life, three of the most common unconscious beliefs we may be doing without realising it are those of hopelessness; "It is hopeless, I can't recover no matter what I do", helplessness; "No one and nothing can help" and worthlessness; "I do not deserve help" or "I cannot reach out for help because that would make me a burden on others".

Do you feel any of these or variations of these?

Even if you logically know that you are worthy of recovery or that other people have recovered and therefore, evidently, recovery is possible, does a part of you still feel that for you it is different?

That's your unconscious beliefs.

Our unconscious beliefs are one of the reasons why we can know so well what to do, have all the information in the world, and still not do it.

A great thing to know is beliefs aren't fact.

They're just one version of reality.

When you truly understand this, everything changes, because imagine what would happen if you didn't have those beliefs.

Imagine if you had a different feeling in their place, a feeling that told you, you could do it. Would that change your actions? Would that change your life?

Beliefs Are Things We Hold to Be True

Attempting to change your beliefs by yourself is complicated because, by definition, beliefs are things we hold to be true.

Can you imagine being able to identify and change something you believe to be the truth? You wouldn't know where to start, and, realistically, you wouldn't even know you had to start, because to you it's truth.

Deep Transformational Change vs. Transient "Understanding"

A beautiful mind is the secret ingredient to a beautiful life.
~ Bonnie Killip

I didn't know I had unconscious beliefs, let alone what they were or that they needed to change if I wanted to live a different way.

It's possible you don't yet either (or it's possible you do know and still feel stuck with how to change them, in which case we'll get to what to do there soon).

I didn't know that my unconscious beliefs were conflicting with my conscious beliefs and preventing me from sustaining recovery, because I wanted recovery so bad! There wasn't anything I wanted more.

It was only when I had help to address my underlying unconscious beliefs that I was finally able to move forward in consistent and sustainable ways.

Until you can get past the barriers created by your unconscious beliefs, any change you manage to make will be transient.

Changing beliefs is one of the things which leads to transformational change, a change that runs so deep it is simply who you now are and is therefore maintained without any effort at all. That's what we're going for in recovery. Every time.

The Very Worst Way of Being Bad

> *I've never seen any life transformation that didn't begin with the person finally getting tired of their own bullshit.*
> *~ Elizabeth Gilbert*

To give you an example of some unconscious beliefs from my own journey, I had one that I could not be a good person without AN.

My unconscious held onto AN as something which allowed me to create the least impact on this world, and as far as I could tell, we needed more of that, with all the climate disasters, animals going extinct, and human corruption.

To be honest, I didn't want to be a part of my own species.

Another unconscious belief my mind held onto was seeing AN as something which gave me immense strength, drive, and determination, something that was always there to push me far beyond my limits and therefore enable me to make great achievements. Achievements I wouldn't be capable of without it.

A part of me believed that without AN, I would be weak and unmotivated. A part of me believed that if I gave up anorexia, I couldn't be there for other people like AN allowed me because I would then be spending time doing what I wanted. Which my unconscious mind at that time believed was selfish, and selfish was the very worst way of being bad.

Those Fears Came to Pass

The greatest weapon against stress is our ability to choose one thought over another.
~ William James.

The truth is many of the things I feared came true. I did make more of an impact on the world, I did stop getting up for predawn marathons, I did stop studying when I wanted to, I did say no to people more often in favour of what I wanted to do.

But, and this is a big "but", none of it meant I was selfish. None of it meant I was a bad person.

I had only believed it meant I was bad, so when I was able to change that belief, doing any of it no longer made me feel bad. None of it now makes me feel bad.

Not because I reasoned it out but because I had help in updating my unconscious beliefs in a way that allowed for those old, fear-based beliefs to simply no longer hold true for me and therefore no longer have any sway over my emotions or life.

Perhaps more importantly, I learnt how to create and connect to a capable self-identity which allows me to know in any circumstance or situation that I am enough, not perfect but enough without question.

5. Developing your Capable Self-Identity

Most of the stress of human beings are emotional ones and the biggest stress of all is trying to be who you are not.
~ Gabor Mate'

Maybe the outside world will eventually change to be exactly as compassionate, kind, understanding, and loving as you want it to be… and maybe it won't. You must ask yourself the question of whether you want to pin your change and your life on the condition of something or someone outside yourself? To recover, you are the only thing you must change. Which is lucky, because you are the only thing you can change.

The Answers to Your Questions are Within You (Only You)

You can't do it through willpower, you have to do it through who you're going to be.
~ Bonnie Killip

You must be doing recovery for you and not for anyone else, because you must be doing life for you.

Until you have developed your strong sense of self, you will be forever swayed by the myriad different and often conflicting messages society is sending you, and you will go nowhere.

It is only when you can stop looking to what other people are doing for a model of what to eat, think, feel, say, or do and look instead within yourself for what to eat, think, feel, say, or do that you will experience what it means to be free.

Who Are You?

Recovery is adapting your mind and actions to the future you want to have not the past you did have.
~ Bonnie Killip

Do you know who you are? How much of your life is yours and how much of your life is ruled by AN?

AN, no matter how much you despise it and how much you don't want it to be true, is an all-invasive illness.

AN becomes a huge part of your identity.

AN, sadly, becomes how other people see you.

It also becomes how you see yourself, so much so that it may now be hard for you to image who or what you would be without it.

However, because the only way to live a life which brings you what you want is to know what you want, and the only way to know what you want is by knowing who you are, you must begin to develop a new self-identity.

You are Not the Behaviour

We are what we repeatedly do. Excellence then, is not an act, but a habit.
~ Will Durant

Many people identify with things or behaviours as inherently them. To give a few suggestions, have you ever heard someone describe themselves as "shy", an "empath", or a "smoker"? These people have come to view these traits (shy or empath) or behaviours (smoking) as very much part of their self-identity. That is; this is who they are.

However, from the outside, we can see that these things are just things they do, not the entirety of who or what they are.

These things we identify as inherently "us" exist at an unconscious level. This is one of the reasons recovery is hard. It is painful for humans to act in ways which are incongruent with their self-identity.

Solution: time to get in touch with your true identity.

Diagnostic Labels Are a Liberation, not a Solution

Make the most of yourself, for that is all there is of you.
~ Ralph Waldo Emerson

Would you be willing to release your attachment to diagnostic labels? Be these labels you or others have placed on you, would you be willing to let them go?

Labels may offer an explanation as to why you are the way you or give validation to what you are experiencing, and in that we can find liberation, but as you now want to be something different, or in the very least not have that label define you entirely, they offer minimal, if any, solutions or guidance on how to be, do, or feel anything different.

What will you have and do without those labels? If not the eating disorder, the anxiety, the depression, the OCD, and so on and so forth, then what?

What will you be without those labels?

Who will you be without those labels?

You Cannot Sacrifice Your Life to Make the Lives of Others Better

Setting an example is not the main means of influencing others, it is the only means.
~ Albert Einstein

Truth: Sacrificing your life does not make the lives of others better. If you run any variation of this martyr script in your head, it's time to let it go. You're not helping anyone or anything by staying small and sick. You can never be sick enough to make someone else healthy, and you can never be sick enough to give someone else a better life.

The only real way to help others is to live your life true to yourself, because this gives others permission to set themselves free and do the same.

Helping anyone else starts with helping you.

Truly helping any other human being starts with healing yourself so you can stop unknowingly and unintentionally perpetuating harm, diet culture, mistrust of our bodies, disconnection, and self-depreciation and instead show what is possible.

Allow yourself a moment to consider this.

Those you respect are they people who've simply given you expert information or told you to do something because it was good for you, or are they people who lived their message? Perhaps they didn't even have to say anything because their genuine and authentic way of being inspired and influenced you.

I know which one it is for me, and I know which one I hold the most admiration and trust for.

Heal Yourself First

Before you can deal with the pain of others, you must first deal with yours.
~ Gabor Mate'

You can't truly promote love and acceptance if you don't practice it in your daily actions toward yourself. The truth always shines through.

You

It's better to be hated for what you are than to be loved for what you are not.
~ Kurt Cobain

The best gift you can share with the world is you.

Living your life to the fullest will make the lives of others infinitely better, because by being you, you can contribute your unique abilities and talents to the world. By being you, you make the world a better place.

It is our highest calling to share with the world all that we are, because we are all incredibly unique, and there are many things that each and every one of us has to contribute that will leave the world a better place for us having lived.

If you stifle this (and AN is an extreme example), then you are denying not only yourself the ability to live to your potential, but you are also denying the world of your magic.

Which brings us to the final area of psychological development and that is giving yourself unconditional permission.

Giving yourself unconditional permission is not a strategy or a tool for success, it is a way of being.

6. Giving Yourself Unconditional Permission

There is overwhelming evidence that the higher the level of self-esteem, the more likely one will be to treat others with respect, kindness and generosity.

~ Nathaniel Branden

Would you be willing to give yourself permission to change? Would you be willing to give yourself permission to be changing?

Would you be willing to give yourself permission to stuff up and keep going?

Would you be willing to give yourself permission to not have it all figured out and to be a work in progress, now and forever?

You Do Not Have to Justify

You yourself, as much as anybody else in the entire universe, deserve your love and affection.
~ Buddha

You do not have to justify eating. You deserve to eat, and that is not conditional on what you ate earlier, what you may eat later, if you hurt someone's feelings, if you think you are going to get a D on your final exam, if you did get a D on your final exam, if you didn't go for that workout, if you forgot to pat your dog goodbye, if you weigh the most you have ever weighed, if others in the world are starving, if there is hatred, unjust, and unspeakable things happening daily, and even if climate change is causing mass devastation around the planet.

You have unconditional permission to eat.

You deserve to eat because you deserve to live and be happy, even in a world where these painful contrasts that shouldn't exist do exist.

You don't just deserve to eat because you are in recovery form an ED, you deserve to eat when you are recovered and healthy.

This is how we live and enjoy life, and you deserve this.

You deserve to eat because you are human.

You Are a Rough and Tumble Human Being, Not A Glass Ornament

> *I began to realise how important it was to be an enthusiast in life. If you are interested in something, no matter what it is, go at it full speed. Embrace it with both arms, hug it, love it, and above all; become passionate about it. Lukewarm is no good.*
> *~ Roald Dahl*

Your life's purpose is not to tip toe around the edges minimizing your probability of experiencing pain.

Your life's purpose is not to walk on eggshells.

Your life's purpose is not to not rock the boat.

Give yourself some credit. You are stronger than that. You are so much stronger than that.

You are not some fragile decoration who needs to be protected from disappointment, heartbreak, or confrontation, you are a human being, and as a human being, you are more than equipped to deal with being let down and with hard experiences.

Certainly, look for pleasure and joy and embrace and fully immerse yourself in those experiences, but at the same time, know that you are incredibly capable of growing through adversity; you were born for it.

Consider giving yourself permission to live.

Life is About More Than You or Me

Be the change you wish to see in the world.
~ Mahatma Ghandi

Most of all, giving yourself unconditional permission comes from knowing life is about more than you or me or even us.

Giving yourself unconditional permission is about recognising that you are human, and it is about having passions and purpose far beyond yourself, living from a place that supports a kind and meaningful world.

Would you be happy to give yourself unconditional permission if it meant you were being a part of supporting a world in which we can all be proud to belong? Because this is exactly what it means.

Conclusion to Psychological Development

There is always more to learn.
~ Bonnie Killip

Recovery will never be a matter of reading a book (regardless of how great) and ticking things one by one off a list in a precise order at a precise time until there are no more things to tick off.

Your recovery is about finding what works for you.

I have done my best to condense a huge topic into these 6 areas, but the reality is they all intertwine as you progress through recovery and life beyond recovery.

In this moment, you may not understand them or see the value in all of them, and that's okay. Leave that to the future you who gets to look back on all the work that you did and decide if it was worth it.

Scary Beyond Necessary is Not Necessary

The difference between despair and hope is the difference between recovery or not.
~ Bonnie Killip

Ultimately, the quality of your life is determined by what you feel and decide it is. Those things that fill you with joy, your passions, purpose, and mission, those things are your choice, not mine and not anyone else's. Your definition of an authentic and fulfilling life is yours alone.

These six areas of psychological development are offerings for you to use as guidelines to bring clarity, direction, and some level of control to your recovery if you so choose.

I offer these as guides because recovery is filled with enough unknowns, and it is undeniably scary and part of that is unavoidable but it doesn't need to be scary beyond what is necessary.

You are Not to Blame

You drown not by falling into a river but by staying submerged in it.
~ Paulo Coelho

While I am focusing on how you will heal yourself with psychological development, I want to be clear that I am not saying your sickness was caused by your lack of psychological development. I am not saying you caused your illness. I am not in any way, shape, or form implying that you should feel guilty.

Please do not confuse cause with cure.

Most illnesses have multiple contributing factors, and AN is no exception. The evidence is in strong support that the development of AN is likely due to a mix of a genetics, environmental conditions and experiences, certain personality "traits", past illness or injury, energy deficit, and stress. None of which you ever had control over. Therefore, you are not to blame for getting sick.

What you do have control over now, however, is your cure.

That does not mean that you can get yourself better simply by willing it so or by thinking or even knowing what to do, because the human brain, and especially a malnourished and sick brain, does not work in this way.

Which is why if you have ever felt stuck with how to change, I encourage you to seek help to learn how to use your mind in new and different ways.

Enter treatment.

Part Four
Treatment

Only when you are happy in who you are can your experience of recovered become stable.
~ Bonnie Killip

4.1 Introduction to Treatment

I know reading this last section on recovery and psychological development may be a lot to take in, and your head may be swimming with how great it all sounds, the excitement and potential of what you want and where you can get to might be inspiring to know, it might also be mixed with trepidation or outright incredulity but any way you're feeling the key question now is "how on earth do I do it?"

How does one cross the unknown and utterly terrifying terrain between where you are and where you want to be?

It's time to find your "how to" get better and beyond.

It is time to find what works for you, because the only reason you haven't made it yet is that you haven't found the right steps for you.

That's all. Nothing more and nothing less complicated than this.

My encouragement is that if you are stuck, it could be time to bring in outside help, which will assist you in taking the steps right for you to first get above the problem, then free of the problem, then develop the skills to ensure it's never a problem again. And, most importantly, it will not only no longer be a problem, but you will have new and more enjoyable, meaningful thoughts, feelings, and behaviours in the place the problem once took up.

The rest of your life needn't be all about focusing on *not* doing something but instead about *doing* something!

Defining Treatment

> *Just because you "should" be able to do it, doesn't mean you can.*
> *~ Bonnie Killip*

To be honest, I don't like to use the word treatment, as it's easy to take it to mean treatment is something being done "to" you or "on" you, and the reality is any meaningful treatment is done "for" you and "with" you.

After deliberation, I decided to go ahead and still use the word "treatment" because I want to draw a distinction between the process of DIY passively hoping it will change or bullying yourself into change "treatment" versus active treatment.

Active Treatment

> *The best preparation for tomorrow is doing your best today.*
> *~ H. Jackson Brown, Jr*

Active treatment is distinct from carrying on telling yourself that it's not that bad, you're not that sick, or making the "battle" or "warrior" mentality part of your identity and the purpose or backbone of your life and identity.

Active treatment is get in and get it done treatment.

This type of treatment includes finding the right outside professional help, because while it is all well and good for me or anyone else to encourage you to seek and accept help, this is only part of the picture. That help really must be the right help for you.

Which is why in this section, it is my intention to clarify some of the different aspects of treatment and your role and rights in it all so you can go in informed and able to make great choices.

After all you are the one that matters most in your treatment.

The Magical Recovery Combination; Care and Know-How

Nothing great was ever achieved without enthusiasm.
~ Ralph Waldo Emerson

I understand if you have trepidation or hesitation toward bringing others into your recovery. Your fears are well founded. I'm not here to convince you otherwise, because you do need to be careful with who you enlist on your recovery team, but what you risk by chancing it alone is far too great.

To recover, and especially to recover quickly, you need people who care, people who are formally educated, have a great understanding of human physiology, nutrition, neurobiology, behaviour, and what it takes to recover from AN.

That is, you need people with that magical combination of both care and know-how.

I Should

Success is not final; failure is not fatal: it is the courage to continue that counts.
~ Winston Churchill

I've been there. I've been in the position of believing I could recover by myself, of believing I *should* recover by myself. I just needed to do what I "knew" I should do—eat.

Having therapist after therapist tell me the same thing or even recommend things which I knew were harmful only reinforced and heightened my frustration, shame, and belief that I was a failure.

"Why can't I just do it!?" "What is wrong with me!?" Were some of my regular thoughts during those years. Perhaps these phrases sound familiar to you?

If you've had a bad experience or bad experiences with treatment, it can be alluring to avoid it altogether, but please do not abandon treatment. There is another option other than trying the very same thing over and over in the desperate hope it works this time.

There is trying something different.

What Do I Look for When Choosing Treatment?

If you do not change direction, you may end up where you are heading.
~ Lao Tzo

Any meaningful treatment needs to work with who you are as a unique individual, because it is ultimately not what the therapist knows that will heal you, it is what you know (even if you don't yet know what you know). Because treatment is always about you.

Most of all, it is you and only you who is in the position to do the hardest part—the doing.

In the end, all (and I really do mean ALL) the credit of your recovery goes to you. This is the way it must be, because if you feel your health is the result of or dependent upon anyone or anything else outside of yourself, you've not found the right help, because the right help will always lead to your empowerment.

A great recovery team will help you with psychological development and empower you to the point where you no longer need their support, because the goal of a recovered life is not to be dependent on your therapist, medication, meditation, or even yoga, friends, family, or the gym, nor anything else to keep you healthy. The goal of recovered is connection to and utter respect and trust in yourself to do the right thing by you without question because it feels good to do so.

Because it wouldn't even entre your mind to not do so.

Because it feels natural to take care of yourself.

You can use all those other things, but the goal of recovery is that they are an adjunct for making your life better and not things you depend on to stay alive.

When to Seek and Accept Help

Yes, you have the rest of your life to figure out recovery,
but wouldn't you rather recover now and simply have the rest of your life?
~ Bonnie Killip

Don't wait for a more convenient time. Don't wait for the epiphany moment. Don't wait to see what happens. Don't wait until you "deserve" help. Don't wait until you have it all figured out. Don't wait until it makes sense. Don't wait until you've given it one more shot alone. Don't wait to get sicker. Don't wait for rock bottom.

Get help today, tonight; make the phone call now, because you will one day look back and understand how sick you really were all those times you thought you weren't "sick enough".

You will one day look back and wonder how on earth you survived, because I can tell you now without a shadow of a doubt that you are far sicker than what you think.

A great way to gauge how sick you are is if you're now thinking you're not sick enough or it's not that bad, because you know what healthy, fully functioning people don't do? They don't settle for "not sick enough". They don't settle for "it's not that bad". What they do is they get help to make it good and great and to constantly improve because they want and deserve good and great, and so do you.

What do you need to seek professional help now?

It's Never Too Soon

> *To improve is to change; to be perfect is to change often.*
> *~ Winston Churchill*

Knowing what I know, if there was just one thing I had the chance to go back in time and change it is that I would seek great treatment sooner and equally that I moved on from treatments that weren't working for me sooner because I did have treatment right from very early on. It just wasn't the treatment for me.

Knowing what I know now, I know there is always a treatment and a way to recover for everyone. It is a shame that I spent so much time sticking out treatments that didn't work for me.

You're allowed to move on from what's not working. Just make sure you keep searching until you find what does work.

In fact, you must, because no one else can do this for you as well as you can. You, more than anyone, know what you need (even if that's someone to help you identify and own what it is you do need).

As hard as it is to step up and say and do what you need, please do it, because you might feel bad about it now, but future you won't have any qualms about your "worthiness". S/he will thank you for you.

Change Requires More than Belief and Motivation

> *Thinking will not overcome fear, but action will.*
> *~ W. Clement Stone*

In my years of illness, there was nothing I wanted more than to get better from AN. There was nothing I fantasised about more than to undo all I felt and to take my brain back to before it changed.

I wanted desperately to be "normal". Yet I couldn't.

The reason why I couldn't change was not a lack of desire, effort, motivation, willpower, or determination, it was that there were and are more ingredients than wanting to change, which are necessary to achieving change.

Ingredients I didn't have. Ingredients I didn't even know I was supposed to have.

Therefore recovered was just a wish, a hope, a dream.

The Three Ingredients for Change

We cannot become what we want by remaining what we are.
~ Max Depree

1. <u>**Want to Change**</u>

Deciding you want to change is crucial to making a deliberate change. But alone, it is not enough.

Please don't waste time getting caught up thinking you just need more motivation or willpower. It's far more likely you have those in abundance. It's far more likely the parts you need to focus on, and which will have a larger impact, are the second two parts of the formula.

2. <u>**Know/Learn How to Change**</u>

The second step, "know how to change", is different to knowing theoretically, because you can know logically what to do (for example eat adequately), but unless you can do it, you don't actually know *how*.

3. <u>**Give Yourself the Chance to Change**</u>

The third step, the chance to change, is a step I think many people skip or cut short when it doesn't go smoothly to plan. And in the real world, it is hard (impossible?) for everything to go precisely to plan.

Your treatment team will provide you with the safe space both mentally and physically where you have the chance to develop all three of these ingredients, and especially the third one, the chance to try out new possibilities.

To me, having a taste of new possibilities is where recovery becomes real.

A Note on Current Treatment

You can't go back and change the beginning, but you can start where you are and change the ending.
~ C. S. Lewis

Having experienced firsthand what the mainstream medical model has to offer people in recovery from AN and having now worked with and heard thousands of other people's stories from across the globe I can quite fairly share that a great deal of people recover in spite of treatment, not because of it.

Losing Some of the Greatest Minds

The treatment many people in recovery from EDs receive is devastating; and without awareness, I don't see how this is going to change.

The more time that passes without changes in treatment is allowing for more people to endure ineffective or even harmful treatment. Which means the higher the cost to the medical system, those suffering, the people who love them, and to the contribution these people would otherwise be making to society and the world.

I honestly believe humanity is losing some of its greatest minds to EDs, and it's all frustratingly needlessly so.

Which is why this area is too important to ignore, and I would not be living in congruency with my values if I were to remain silent on this.

Hospitalisation is Not Recovery

Currently, our medical system works off an acute care model, where patients are hospitalised, partially weight restored, and discharged when they are no longer considered at high medical risk.

I don't want to overlook the fact that this is entirely necessary. It is lifesaving. However, what I've come to realise is that while the treatment in hospital is necessary and lifesaving, how the treatment in hospital is delivered and the follow up is where we have far to go.

Hospitalisation experiences are frequently traumatic, and discharge often comes with no support or clear plan on where to go to from here in terms of connection to or offering of further treatment options. Which means the whole ordeal leaves people reeling. They leave feeling abused, deserted, confused, unheard, uncared for, and utterly untrusting toward health professionals and what treatment and recovery mean.

All of which unfortunately further erodes faith in the world's ability to help and your ability to heal.

From this perspective, it is easy to understand why people living with EDs frequently end up in hospital again and again (and again and again).

It has nothing to do with getting out of hospital and being determined to lose the weight you gained (as a textbook would have you believe) and everything to do with the fact that weight gain (partial or "full") is not, never has been, and never will be a cure for AN.

Fundamentally Misinformed

The favourite word in classic definitions of AN is "refusal". With "Refusal to gain weight" and "refusal to eat" being up there amongst the most common phrases used to describe AN. Each of which implies that not eating is an act of freewill (that it is the choice of the person with AN to either eat or not eat). This is what health professionals are taught. Which means that unless they've had firsthand experience themselves or with someone they love living with an ED, this is what they believe.

This is where the treatment of AN becomes more harmful than helpful, because this means people who are in positions to treat those in recovery from AN are profoundly misinformed.

People with AN are being treated from a fundamentally flawed concept of what the illness is, which means there is little room for progress from here.

Disempowerment

Treatment from such a mindset that the person with AN is acting out of freewill or that they are devious, manipulative, or flat out liars insists on taking the control out of the hands of the sufferer, because from this view, they are "incompetent" and just need to stop harming themselves.

We condense a human being to an illness, and from here it's impossible to establish any semblance of the type of therapeutic relationship necessary for recovery.

When I was sick, I was surprised and hurt every time I was treated as though I didn't want to get better.

I was possibly one of the most rule abiding, compliant, and eager to recover patients to ever exist.

What I realise now is that hospital staff were not adequality trained in what AN is and how to care for someone with this illness, let alone help them move them forward.

They only understood it as a battle against the person.

The saddest thing is that when you are sick with AN, you do not have the mental stability or resilience to cope in such an environment, and rather than recognising it's a downfall of the system, it comes across as personal. It comes across as blame. While this is not the intention, it doesn't make the effects any less devastating.

There is nothing more confusing, nothing more perpetuating of the illness nor more damaging, than being treated as though you are the problem. You already believe that.

You Can't Force Recovery Upon Someone

What is necessary to change a person is to change his awareness of himself.
~ Abraham Maslow

You can't force recovery upon someone, because you can't force someone to be healthy. You can force the things we associate with treatment, for example, nasogastric tubes (NGs) or meal replacement drinks and so on, and I can see how it is tempting to do so, but this is not recovery. This is not recovery because it does not set the foundations for this person to trust themselves and to survive out there in the world to the best of their capabilities. It teaches the opposite and reinforces that they cannot and should not trust their own body. That they are incompetent and cannot survive out there in the world on their own.

Threats Are Archaic

Only in the presence of compassion will people allow themselves to see the truth.
~ Gabor Mate'

Threats, force, or blame with the intention of getting someone to eat are archaic. To be honest, it says more about the misconceptions of society and the people delivering these forms of "treatment" than anything else.

Cling on or Drown

If we continuously try to force a child to do what he is afraid to do, he will become more timid and will use his brains and energy not to explore the unknown but to find ways to avoid the pressures put upon him.
~ John Holt

The principal that threats and forceful exorcism works off of is a well-meaning one because it is intended that if the ED behaviours are taken away, you will learn to swim.

Indeed, this may be the case for a healthy person (maybe), but AN is an illness, and the person is not healthy. The brain and abilities of someone with AN are not those of a healthy person. They have no other ways of coping. They have no other options, because they have no other way of being (yet).

Therefore, the reality of the outcome of this form of "treatment" is that they either cling on more tightly to the illness or drown, because until they know how to let go, they can't let go.

It's not a choice.

Post Traumatic Growth

There are many experiences in life which words cannot bring justice to, and hospitalisation with AN is one of them.

If you have had a bad hospital experience, from the bottom of my heart, I am truly sorry.

The truth may be that hospitalisation is lifesaving. It saved my life. On more than one occasion. But it was also some of the most traumatic experiences of my life.

While I cannot undo what has been done and the pain you have been through, I can help you become stronger than it.

Post traumatic growth, where the person after a traumatic experience (including the years of abuse at the hands of an ED or being hospitalised) recovers and goes on to live the rest of their life at a higher level of strength and success than had they not had the traumatic experience, is as real a phenomenon as post-traumatic stress disorder (PTSD).

You are the only one who can choose to survive and thrive even after all the messed-up things that shouldn't have happened, happened.

A Better Way

Don't Find Fault, Find A Remedy.
~ Henry Ford

It is never my intention to point out what is wrong with treatment and leave it at that. It is my intention to provide a clear way of doing things better and be a part of advocating for and delivering better.

Shifting the Focus to Where it's Needed

When we switch from focusing on the problem to focusing on the solution, everything changes.
~ Bonnie Killip

I want to make it abundantly clear that I am not beating up the medical system. I am a part of the medical system, and it is not only necessary but also wonderful. There is no question that medical intervention is often necessary in recovery, but it must come hand in hand with psychological development if it is to be anything more than a means of prolonging life.

You've likely experienced that none of the strictly medical procedures have cured you yet. Not the IVs, the NG tubes, the heart monitors, iron infusions, B12 shots, the constant weighing, BGL checking, nor the BP monitoring. None of these procedures will make you recover.

Make full use of all medical resources available to you, including regularly seeing your doctor for monitoring and evaluation of your physical health, because you are at high risk of many physiological problems, and this is your doctor's area of expertise.

No amount of psychological development will protect you from the physical implications of malnutrition and starvation but be realistic on the fact that their purpose is not to cure.

Hospitals are not designed and were never designed for psychological recovery from an eating disorder, and without psychological recovery, there is no recovery. This is not a judgement; it is a fact, and when you realise and accept this, you can put your efforts and energy into finding the treatment you do need.

Challenging the Status Quo

The best fighter is never angry.
~ Lao Tzu

I acknowledge that there will be people who will disagree with my treatment recommendations, and I welcome and expect this, because they are different. They are not the status quo. However, the number of people developing EDs is increasing, the recovery rates from EDs are not increasing, and the so called "gold standards" of ED treatment are failing spectacularly.

Therefore, perhaps it is time someone did challenge the status quo. Evidently, new approaches to treatment are needed.

The Way It Is Rather than the Way It Should Be

Nothing changes if nothing changes.
~ Janet Gwen

It was never my intention to write a book designed purely to keep all happy. If I were to do so, it wouldn't hold much value for those I am writing to serve. You.

My heart, energy, and loyalties lie firmly with those still suffering. To whom I would be doing a monumental disservice if I were to remain silent or share only information of the way it should be rather than the way it is.

If Only They'd Do What I Say!

If everyone continues to skirt around the issue that treatment is failing or insist treatment is failing because the patient doesn't want to get better, isn't ready, or, worst of all, that if only they'd follow the advice, they'd be fine, then people will continue to suffer. People will continue to die.

If blame continues to be put on the person in recovery, then healing is only going to be delayed or prevented entirely. I do not want this, because everyone who lives with an ED is ready to recover. Certainly, they can be very afraid to live another way, believe they are incapable of living another way, believe they are unworthy of living another way, or not know how to live another way, but none of these are the same as not wanting or not being ready to recover.

While I know I got the help I needed eventually, and I am abundantly grateful for this, the time that I missed out on, the time I spent in uncertainty and fear, is time I can never, ever get back.

I don't wish this for you. I don't wish this for anyone else.

Change the System Slowly and Lives Now

A man can fail many times, but he isn't a failure until he begins to blame somebody else.
~ John Burroughs

I advocate for change at the system level while also at the same time work with people in recovery from EDs directly and outside of the larger systems. I am not going to wait for the system to change. I am not going to wait for the system to change when I can be one of those offering an alternative by helping individuals gain freedom and live their lives now.

It was one person, just one person out of numerous people I sought help from, who helped me change my life.

It can be one person who helps you change your entire existence. Find them.

Get Great Help, Get Well

Make this not just the end of something awful but the beginning of something amazing.
~ Bonnie Killip

As you've been reading this book, and this section in particular, I hope you have gained an appreciation of how much the people involved in your treatment or the treatment of your loved one truly do matter. If you appreciate this, then I encourage you to become an active participant in ensuring that you get the help you need or help your loved one to find the help they need and to step up and put this in place for them if they are holding back.

Your loved one is stuck. They are not "resisting" treatment because they want to stay sick but because their self-worth combined with the illness will not allow it.

Please consider investing in them. Please consider showing them they are more than worthy, because then they will get better, and you can stop living this nightmare alongside them.

Make this not just the end of something awful but the beginning of something amazing.

Don't Complicate It

Start by doing what's necessary; then do what's possible; and suddenly you are doing the impossible.
~ Francis of Assisi

I did not recover because I had the perfect environment and support to recover. I did not recover because I was "ready". I did not recover by accident. It didn't just happen. I did not recover because there was anything special about me. I recovered because of one thing and one thing only.

I found the help I needed.

Which means had I not, I would right now in this very moment, without a shadow of a doubt, be in the midst of just holding on or fighting my way out of yet another relapse.

That, or dead.

Continuing that path, these were my only realistic options, and that's a powerful thing to know and exactly why I am so passionate about sharing practical suggestions for treatment options, because while there is always the possibility they may not work for you, there is equally also the possibility they may.

Who Makes Up My Power Recovery Team?

I have decided to stick with love. Hate is too great a burden to bear.
~ Martin Luther King

To tell you the truth, when I wrote the first copy of this book, I was angry. I was angrier than I've ever been in my entire life, and it was a very different book because of this.

I was mad and so deeply hurt because I had been let down by not only the bureaucratic protocol of the "system", but also, as much as I didn't want to believe it, didn't want to acknowledge it, and certainly didn't want to say it out loud; undeniably, very much so by the individuals involved in my "treatment".

I vehemently wanted to protect others in the vulnerable position I had been in from ever going through what I had gone through, and to me, this meant connecting them with the exact kind of help I had found and which changed it all for me.

However, I now know the people who will help you heal are those who will help you heal. I now know your power team are who you choose because your recovery is in your hands.

There are many paths that lead to recovered, and it comes down to finding what works for you.

When I was sick, I saw people with great long lists of credentials and years of experience and expertise that "should" have helped me heal but didn't. Couldn't. I also now know people with the very same credentials on paper as the person who did help me heal and who wouldn't have been able to help me heal had I seen them instead. There's more to it than credentials or experience. People are people.

Which is why your power team comprises those who are of most help to you. It is only you who can truly make that choice. Therefore, while I am about to provide suggestions on what a Power Recovery Team may look like, you must pick and choose or find your own entirely new path, because, ultimately, the only right way to recover is the way that works for you.

That is the path of recovery, learning to live for you.

4.2 Introducing the Power Recovery Team

The only place where success comes before work is in the dictionary.
~ Vidal Sassoon

In the following pages, I will be sharing my treatment recommendations based on my personal experience of recovery from AN as well as my professional experience helping others recover from AN, binge eating disorder, bulimia nervosa, avoidant restrictive food intake disorder (ARFID), and everything across, around, within, and outside the spectrum of what weird and wonderful things human beings can do with food and their bodies.

There are three core competences and characteristics people must have in order to fulfill my criteria of a Power Recovery Team. This can be one person, or it can be twenty people.

Firstly, an ED Dietitian or someone with expert knowledge in human biology, health, and nutrition with a specific interest in what it takes to recover from an ED.

Secondly, a Neurolinguistic Programming (NLP) and Clinical Hypnotherapy practitioner or someone who understands neurobiology and how the human brain works at an unconscious level. Also, preferably with expertise in how this applies to recovery from an ED.

Thirdly, a skilled and professionally trained coach. Again, ideally with expertise in ED recovery.

Openly Biased

Experience is knowledge. All the rest is information.
~ Albert Einstein

I am a Dietitian, I am a clinical and medical hypnotherapist, I am a neurolinguistic programming practitioner, and I am a life and success coach; therefore, I am biased on all three of the credentials I recommend as being core to your Power Recovery Team.

However, there is one reason why I have trained in these and why I will continue to do so, and that reason is because they work.

I truly believe that these are the skills necessary for someone or more than one person on your recovery team to possess in order for you to recover faster than you may think possible, and perhaps necessary for you to recover at all.

Why do I think this? Because I was in recovery for fifteen years. This did not mean that for fifteen years I was slowly getting better. It meant for fifteen years I was sick. Very sick.

It meant I spent fifteen years of my life shamefully shuffling into and out of various therapists' offices, being wheelchaired into and out of a never-ending procession of hospitals literally the world over, all the while broken and afraid and always on the verge of giving up.

It meant fifteen years of my life was ruled by confusion, shame, fear, crippling self-doubt, anxiety, depression, addictions, and uncertainty.

It meant for fifteen years, my daily life was thinking, feeling, and doing things I did not want to be thinking, feeling, or doing.

That is fifteen years, or 5299 days, or 126,176 hours, or 7,630,560 minutes, or 457, 833, 6000 seconds of my life I will never get back.

And I am one of the lucky ones. I made it through alive. I recovered, and to have a chance at a recovered life is nothing short of a miracle, with what my mind, body, and soul went through, yet it needn't have been so.

So, if you think I am biased in my recommendations, yes, I am. Openly, unapologetically, loudly, and happily so, because my interest is no longer in "not rocking the boat" it is in helping those still suffering gain freedom as soon as possible.

This is your one precious chance at life.

Overview of Your Power Recovery Team

The secret of change is to focus all your energy, not on fighting the old but on building the new.
~ Socrates

In this section, it is my intention to provide you with a brief overview of each of the professions I recommend you seek when building your recovery team—Dietetics, Clinical Hypnotherapy and Neurolinguistic Programming (which I am counting together, and you will soon see why), and Coaching.

Please know this really is a short introduction to these fields, and there is much more to each than I could possibly hope to cover here. This section is by no means designed to be a comprehensive guide to their intricacies, it is merely an offering of what else is available.

Therefore, without further ado, I welcome you to the first of the three skills I'd highly recommend you look for when choosing your team.

1. Dietitian

Man cannot remake himself without suffering, for he is both the marble and the sculptor.
~ Alexis Carrel

Why a Dietitian?
I learnt there was such a thing as a Dietitian when I found myself sitting in the waiting room for my first appointment with a dietitian. I was around thirteen years old at the time. I was starved and malnourished. I didn't know what was happening. I didn't know I was sick. I truly didn't understand that I wasn't eating enough. I didn't know how much you were supposed to eat. I had lost all ability to self-regulate my food intake. I didn't want to believe you had to eat. I don't remember much of that visit,

nor the visits to follow. However, what I do know is it was thanks to that dietitian that my life was saved.

This dietitian (who later became one of my supervisors when I went through my university dietetics training many years later and who is now an inspiring friend) helped my parents to understand how much food it would take for me to regain weight and physical health.

For her expertise that went into developing and delivering the "diet plan" she prescribed and the permission to eat she gave, I am infinitely grateful.

For her unwavering certainty and consistency, I am even more grateful, because my uncertain, starved, stressed, and overwhelmed mind needed that steady confidence.

I used the outline of this same meal plan each time I relapsed (which was numerous times in the years that would follow) as "permission" to eat, and each time it would enable me to regain weight.

Evidently, it wasn't a cure, or I'd have not needed to keep coming back to this meal plan for so long. So, what was missing? Why didn't it "fix me?" I was missing the psychological treatment alongside the refeeding. I believe had I had the psychological treatment I found years later at the same time as the support and expertise of this dietitian, I have no doubt I'd have recovered immediately.

Anorexia was never necessary in my life. Just as it's not in yours.

The Stakes are Your Life

In recovery, the stakes are not just high; the stakes are your life.

Recovery from AN is not a time for wishy-washy guidance or people just giving it a go, which means the people who are offering input into your recovery must be competent to give you the right information. You shouldn't even be considering putting your life into the hands of anyone less than expert level. This is especially true when it comes to the nutrition and food side of recovery, because the only thing which will heal you physically is food (and rest).

A Dietitian Is a Nutrition Expert

Fad diets are usually suggested or supported by professionals who have little or no training in evidence-based nutrition.
~ Mpho Tshukudu

A dietitian is the only health professional I would recommend seeking dietary advice from during recovery.

Dietitians have completed a four-year university degree or a couple of years of masters and another year of mentorship and obligatory ongoing annual professional development and training in food science, nutritional biochemistry, and human health. There is no equivalent.

Advice from anyone else, no matter how well recognised their credentials as a health professional, is a risk.

Specialising in Eating Disorders

Nutrition is the missing ingredient in mental health treatment.
~ Bonnie Killip

When choosing a dietitian, you must choose someone who works with people in recovery from EDs. Preferably someone who has recovered from an eating disorder. The reason for this is twofold; first of all, they will be able to better psychologically support you, but also, they need to be trained in the nutritional requirements for someone recovering from an ED.

Without additional training and interest in the treatment of people with EDs, it would be easy to under prescribe a dietary plan. Which at the very least will never get you to full recovery and at the most is life-threatening.

How A Dietitian Can Help

We are indeed much more than what we eat, but what we eat can nevertheless help us to be much more than what we are.
~ Adelle Davis

In the early stages of recovery, I highly encourage you to follow a meal plan. This is something I've put considerable thought into, and after revisiting this section of this book with the intention of changing this recommendation multiple times, I've solidly decided to keep it in.

Why did I think about taking it out? Because more than anything, recovery from an ED is about learning how to trust your body and to give it what it needs. This cannot come from a meal plan. Not even the world's best meal plan.

However, why I have decided to continue advocating for a meal plan in the beginning of recovery is because I see the real-life results of well-meaning attempts to do intuitive eating before these skills are developed (or rather redeveloped, because we are all born with these skills).

Hence, I know it would be unrealistic, detrimental, and dangerous to advocate listening to your body's cues as a first step of recovery. It isn't realistic.

The fact is, you will need to eat a substantial amount of food regularly and for far longer than you think.

The goal of eating in recovery is not "normal eating". It is overeating.

A plan is the best way to ensure you meet your needs when you are not comfortable eating to your hunger or don't yet know how to eat to your hunger. And if you are in recovery from an eating disorder, you meet those criteria.

What is an Eating Plan?

Proper nutrition is the key to unlock your body's potential.

~ Brian Holifield

An eating plan is a meal plan you've cocreated with your Dietitian.

The amount of food or additional energy you need to eat will be unique to you, but to give you an idea of what some of the literature out there is saying, studies cite the need for a range anywhere between 12,000kJ (4,000cal) to 48,000kJ (12,000cal) additional kilojoules (additional means above what it would take for you to maintain weight) per week to gain approximately a kilogram of weight per week.

However, most recognise, and it was certainly my personal experience, that it is often substantially more than this due to numerous factors, including decreased absorptive capacity of your GI tract and if you are doing any exercise.

On a personal note, I ate in excess of 18,800kJ or 4500cal consistently day in and day out for well over a year to restore weight. However, this was motivated from a place of fear of losing weight. When recovery truly became a possibility was when I surrendered. I just ate and ate and ate as a full-time commitment.

It was when I let go of the meal plan and the numbers and the trying to get it right that recovery changed, but it was only because of the safety the meal plan had initially provided that I was able to get into a position where I was ready to let go of the meal plan!

The Value of a Meal Plan

Courage, cheerfulness and a desire to work depends mostly on good nutrition.
~ Jacob Moleschott

Having a meal plan can help lessen the indecision over what to eat and when to eat. It is pre-decided which is incredibly valuable in the early stages of recovery when the thought of making food decisions is overwhelming.

Having something reliable to follow that allows you to eat is key to physical and psychological repair, because adequate and consistent nutrition is the foundation of physical and psychological wellbeing for all of us, not just those in recovery from AN.

What you eat gives you energy, and without energy you won't be able to do the work to recover and more importantly to create and live an enjoyable and fulfilling life by any definition.

On a biological level, following a meal plan allows the emotional centres of your mind to be soothed and feel safe, and it is only from a place of safety that you'll begin to feel ready to address the challenge of change.

When you are well nourished, your brain is able to process things you cannot process when your body is concerned only with surviving. This isn't personal. It's mammal. It's human.

A food plan can give you part of the safety and certainty.

Ideally, I would encourage you to take someone with you for your initial dietetics consultation. This could be this your carer, parents, partner, friend, or other, because it is important that others in your life know how much food is required for you to eat to gain health. Not so they can enforce or police your intake but so they can be aware, because this practical side of recovery is out of the realm of their knowledge.

Postpone the Judgement

People are very open-minded about new things as long as they're exactly like the old ones.
~ Charles F. Kettering

You might think you know what to eat, that whatever the dietitian tells you to eat you can't eat anyway, they don't understand, or they're going to tell you the wrong things to eat or make you eat too much or too little, but even with all those thoughts, consider making the appointment and making the value judgement later.

You don't need to understand how they can help you in this moment for them to help in this moment.

You'll Need More

Food is an important part of a balanced diet.
~ Fran Lebowitz

What the dietitians I saw during my recovery unfortunately did not have (because I saw a few) were the skills to help me to change the thought patterns and the reasons why eating was so hard for me.

Frustratingly, it took me many, many more years to find someone who could help me change my thought patterns, feelings, and behaviours, and this is where I simply cannot recommend a Neurolinguistic Programming (NLP) and Clinical Hypnotherapy practitioner enough (or a dietitian that operates using all these tools).

Why? Because both NLP and Hypnotherapy are about the doing. They are concerned with "how to" change.

Whereas the traditional and more conservative forms of psychiatry, psychology, and psychotherapy I experienced were focused on what was wrong and exploring and exposing why and where it may have gone wrong. All with the underlying thread that talking about the problem or understanding why it had happened would spontaneously lead to recovery.

Spoiler alert: it didn't.

I am not disregarding the importance of talking about the problems, stresses, and what's happening in your life; however, the difference is, when you are in recovery from an ED and desperate for change, all the talking in the world is not going to produce that change.

There are plenty of people who understand why they are doing whatever problem it is that they are doing, and yet they are still living with that problem.

When you're free of the problem and your brain is no longer controlled by fear, then talking is useful. Then talking is amazing, because you can use it, but when you are so far below and consumed by the problem, talking isn't going to cut it.

So, who can help you get out of the problem?

2. Clinical Hypnotherapist and Neurolinguistic Programming Practitioner

Peace cannot be kept by force; it can only be achieved by understanding.
~ Albert Einstein

Doing Everything "Right"
At thirteen, my body was shutting down. At fourteen, I was pulled out of school. At fifteen, I felt like the most alone person in the world.

I was perpetually cold, my long hair almost completely fell out, my skin became dry, sunken, and yellow-greyish, my teeth wobbled in my gums, my eyes hurt, and my bones ached every time I sat still.

In the years to come, my life became a series of expeditions in and out of hospital and seeing what felt like an endless procession of doctors, dietitians, and therapists.

My days literally revolved around food, medical monitoring, and psychological "treatment" (as well as the huge amounts of schoolwork I insisted on doing).

Theoretically, I was doing recovery right, but rather than move through it and out the other side, this quasi-recovery became my life.

I spent fifteen years living with anorexia before I had a taste of what else was possible. That introduction came in the form of clinical hypnotherapy and NLP. Two modalities that helped me learn to truly use my mind (a mind that by that time I despised) in new ways.

Why an NLP and Clinical Hypnotherapy Practitioner?

> *When you get people out of their normal mode of thinking it's pretty easy to do new things.*
> *~ Richard Bandler*

Nutritional renourishment will get you so far, understanding the components of psychological development will get you further.

Yet it is the conviction and belief that you can live not only without the ED but with things which are far more meaningful in its place which matters most.

Conviction is what ensures your transformation is lifelong rather than a moment of intellectual insight.

It is hypnotherapy and NLP which speed up and may even be necessary to make this possible because they work at the only level where change will lead to lasting change; the level of your unconscious.

You Have More to Gain Than Freedom from Pain

> *Happiness is a way of travel not a destination.*
> *~ Roy Goodman*

I was incredibly fortunate that in 2017 my mum gave me a newspaper clipping that was given to her by my dad, who was in turn given it by my grandma or something like that. I'm unclear on the origin.

This newspaper clipping was of a story about a woman (who has since become a friend) who had recovered from AN.

I had not long been discharged from what I can only describe as a particularly horrific hospital experience and was in the throes of force-feeding myself to gain weight to be "healthy", or rather to never go back to hospital again.

Yet again.

At that stage, I can confidently say I did not believe in full recovery. I had all but resigned myself to a best-case scenario of a lifetime of "maintenance". A lifetime of forcing myself to eat, to tenuously hold on to some semblance of physical "health".

I didn't believe I'd ever be mentally well.

In any case, there was no way I could have conceived of a greater concept for my future than lessening the pain.

I certainly didn't yet know that I had anything to gain.

One Question to Change It All

The greatest discovery of all time is that a person can change his future by merely changing his attitude.
~ Oprah Winfrey

I called the woman from the paper and asked her one question.

How? An incredulous, and I will admit entirely sceptical, "how on earth did you recover?"

She told me that she had one person instrumental in her recovery, a woman who practised hypnotherapy and something called Neurolinguistic Programming (NLP).

The first (hypnosis), I did not believe in, coming from a heavily scientific background, or at least did not see it as something that would work "on" me, maybe on others, but certainly not me.

The second (NLP), I had never even heard of. It didn't sound promising.

But I had run out of alternatives.

Everything that had sounded promising, everything that was supposed to have helped, had failed.

Down the Rabbit Hole

Most people walk through this world in a trance of disempowerment.
Our work is to transform that into a trance of empowerment.
~ Milton Erickson

It was my mum who booked my first hypnotherapy appointment, because I didn't feel worthy to spend money on myself.

It felt like a waste.

I still held the belief that I could and should get better on my own because it was simple; just eat. It was so far from rocket science it wasn't funny. People did it naturally every day. Two-year-old children were out there doing it without a thought.

I didn't want to pay for more people to tell me to eat. I was acutely and ashamedly aware that was a problem.

I turned up terrified on that first day. I turned up ready to reopen all the wounds and rehash all the traumas. I turned up ready to quietly share my shame, self-hate and disappointment at my own stupidity through tears and snot while yet another therapist scrutinised, judged, and attempted to logic and reason me into some kind of behavioural change. That, or sought to lump blame on me, my parents, my school, my friends, or society for my problem, leaving me feeling more ashamed, pathetic, crazy and with even less clue how to change anything than before I had walked in.

Fortunately, and to my relief, that was not how the sessions went.

There was still much crying and snot in the initial sessions, because talking about myself was exceptionally uncomfortable, and the sessions were exhausting. But they were exhausting in a different way to what I'd experienced before. In a way that was useful. In a way that opened my brain to new ways of thinking, not just as a nice concept or something which made sense intellectually yet was frustratingly unobtainable, but as a real choice.

Hypnosis does not remove choice, it gives you choice so that way you're feeling or that thing you're doing which you don't want to be feeling or doing becomes just one of many options available to you at any time rather than your only option.

One Moment to Change It All

Be happy for this moment, this moment is your life.
~ Omar Khayyam

That first consult was truly the moment my recovery became recovery versus being sick, knowing I was sick and wanting to be recovered.

I honestly owe my life to this one woman.

Not because she did it for me, not because she was empathetic or caring or an expert on AN, or any other ED for that matter, and not because she got me better, but because she put in the effort to learn the skills (clinical hypnotherapy, NLP, and professional coaching), and more importantly, I believe she put in the work to consistently be the person who could help.

She was the role model and inspiration I trusted and respected (and which I'd not found anywhere else in my life).

The Liberation of Choice

The best way to predict your future is to create it.
~ Abraham Lincoln

For the first time ever, I had choices. For the first time ever, I could see and feel what I could do to change in this moment; not what I could do to change at some unspecified future date, but now.

For the first time ever, I had the belief that I could change. For the first time ever, I had a future.

I didn't just understand that I had choices, I felt I had choices. I believed I had choices. I knew I had choices.

I believed that the way I thought and behaved was under my control to change, and I knew I was capable of making those changes irrespective of anyone or anything that had influenced and held me back in the past, and, amazingly, I did.

Even more amazingly, they began to feel normal(ish).

They now feel normal.

They weren't easy decisions and the actions certainly were far from a breeze but I now know the certainty I was looking for, that I often see my clients seeking only exists in hindsight.

Life Creating

This was not just lifechanging, it was life creating.

I felt, rather than imagined or longed after, a new way of living, and the two cannot be compared.

What Are Hypnotherapy and NLP?

Words don't teach, experience does.
~ Bonnie Killip

Hypnotherapy and NLP are ways by which we can help someone who has not been able to change through consciously trying to change.

You can talk logically about your problem for an hour, the next two months, a year, five years, thirty-five years, or the rest of your life, and you may gain some level of understanding, clarity, or relief each time you do this, but often that is it.

With an ED, you'll often find you're not going to truly generate solutions or get anywhere by talking, because your conscious, logical mind isn't the part doing the problem. You don't have a conscious problem. But you do have an unconscious problem.

AN exists at the unconscious level. It's not intellectual. You, therefore, cannot reason or willpower your way out of it.

Rather than lament this, NLP and hypnotherapy offer a tangible means of utilising this. Essentially, NLP and clinical hypnotherapy are both tools for updating old and unwanted neural pathways with new, more desirable ones. They do this by working with our physiology and unconscious mind rather than our conscious mind.

In truth, they work with both, but their impact on the unconscious mind is what sets them apart from other forms of therapy and which allows for a level of fast and lasting change that very possibly simply cannot be achieved consciously.

Utilising the Unconscious Mind for Change

You must expect great things of yourself before you can do them.
~ Michael Jordan

Up until about the 1800s, therapy had largely been dominated by rational talking it out type therapy based on the premise that understanding why and where the problem came from combined with empathy and guidance from the therapist would lead to change.

This method didn't always succeed, and people looked for more.

Two new ways of understanding human behaviour entered the scene. One of which was hypnosis and the other evolutionary biology. Both hypnosis and evolutionary biology acknowledge and make use of the fact that not all behaviours can be explained rationally or changed through rational understanding alone.

Both recognise the presence of an "unconscious" mind.

It is not too difficult to describe hypnotherapy and NLP from a theoretical or scientific level, but because NLP and hypnotherapy are both tools of experience, words will never truly capture what they allow for in terms of the change in someone's life, including my own life, because for that, I can tell you, there are no words.

Recovery requires changing your automatic thought processes, those which are preventing you from feeling and acting in ways which support your health, happiness, and fulfillment, and this can only be done at a level deeper than conscious awareness, because that is where your automatic responses arise.

If you or anyone else are wanting to create any long-term change, it must eventually move from conscious desire and learning to unconscious control.

Fundamental health sustaining activities such as sleeping and eating should largely be generated from your unconscious. It's very difficult to consciously make yourself sleep. Just as it is very difficult to consciously know what and how much to eat. Eating is an unconscious process that has become conscious in people living with EDs but which never should have.

Health is Your Default

I am sure you've heard the word "homeostasis" before. This is essentially a state of perpetually striving for balance and health. Your body's natural and inbuilt functions are all geared toward creating homeostasis.

Your body is on your team. At an unconscious level, your body is determinedly and competently steering you toward health twenty-four hours a day, seven days a week, and it does this without your micromanagement. In fact, it does this largely without your conscious awareness at all and certainly without your conscious effort.

Healthy is not something you have to force yourself to be, it is not something you have to trick, motivate, or hack your body into doing, because it is something your body naturally both wants and knows exactly how to do.

To support health, all you must do is supply your body with the tools and step out of the way. It will always do what is best for you, because this is what it is designed to do.

Your level of health may be different to others and may look different to others, but your body is on your team. Your body literally has no other choice or intention than to do it's best by you.

Stop Downplaying Your Pain

Turn your wounds into wisdom.
~ Oprah Winfrey

Experiencing NLP and hypnotherapy are hands down what I attribute my entire recovery to. Without hypnotherapy and NLP, I can honestly say that I don't think I would have healed. I was so stuck.

The more I wanted to be "normal", the more it seemed impossible. The more I fought with myself and tried to shut out, avoid, ignore, or downplay the things which hurt me, the more I suffered.

Hypnosis and NLP gave me a means of learning how to get out of the way and let my body do what it knew how to do all along.

Easier Does Not Mean Less Powerful

Time doesn't heal you; you heal you.
~ Bonnie Killip

AN is a multifaceted and complex illness, and there is no denying that recovery is difficult, but I don't believe it need be as difficult, traumatic, or as long as conventional treatment would have us believe.

There may be simpler ways to recover than anyone has shared with you, and simpler does not mean they are any less powerful. Recovery is recovery, whether it takes you one month or twenty-two and three quarters of a year. There are no awards for recovering slower and there are no reasons why a longer recovery is any better, more thorough, or real. Quick change is possible, humans do it all the time.

NLP and hypnotherapy are tools which facilitate change at a pace more rapidly and more completely than anything I have yet experienced because they were created through real life experience and modelling what works.

Not a Logical Problem

The less effort the more powerful you will become.
~ Bruce Lee

AN is not a logical problem. Therefore, all the reasoning, rationalising, and exploring ways to eat more in a therapist's office where it's safe and secure to do so won't lead to it feeling okay out there in your real life.

You have probably experienced some variation of this, whether it be the pep talk you, a doctor, a therapist, family member, partner, or someone else gives you and which sounds great and reasonable at the time but when you go out into the real world, into the context of your everyday life, it doesn't stand up.

You fail time and time again.

You fail no matter how many of these rational, meaningful, inspiring, promising, motivating, or threatening talks you construct or receive, because when it comes to the situation, your rational mind is nowhere to be found.

Out there, in your real life where it matters most, because your life is lived in the real world, not the therapy room, all that logical stuff you talked about and which made so much sense often feels less than useless. Other than the fact you can then use it to beat yourself up over your failings, because how could you be so stupid?

When, in actuality, it has nothing to do with your intelligence, willpower, or motivation and everything to do with looking for the answer in the wrong place.

No Matter How Thoroughly You Look, if it's in the Wrong Place, You Won't Find It

A man saw Nasrudin searching for something on the ground. "What have you lost, Mulla?" he asked. "My key," said the Mulla.

So, they both went down on their knees and looked for it.

After a time, the other man asked: "Where exactly did you drop it?"

"In my house."

"Then why are you looking here?"

"There is more light here than inside my house."

My NLP and Hypnotherapy Walk on the Wild Side

In order to gain possession of ourselves we have to have some confidence, some hope of victory, in order to keep that hope alive we must usually have some taste of victory we must know what victory is and like it better than defeat.
~ *Thomas Merton*

Once I began looking in the right place, I began making change. Often without even being aware that I was.

Those things which once destroyed me and which I believed were out of my hands I was suddenly not bothered by, and I mean suddenly, because after fifteen years of daily inner turmoil and struggle, I was finally starting to have choice and therefore make changes.

I am talking profound, life-changing results, not transient feel better for a moment, an hour, or a day type "results".

What was revolutionary for me was that, unlike all the intellectual reasoning I'd bullied myself with in the years prior, these results didn't disappear when things got tough.

I was becoming increasingly empowered, which meant I was able to increasingly gain evidence that I could, in fact, do it.

I was no longer spending "therapy" sessions shamefully discussing all the ways in which I'd failed and all the ridiculous easy things I still couldn't do and how hopeless I was or lying about how I was making progress because I was too ashamed to admit I still couldn't do that thing we'd talked about doing for the past three years.

Instead, I was stepping into my power and proving that I could do it because, ultimately, how we change our lives is through experience.

Experience is proof.

To know and believe that the life you are recovering into is going to be "worth it" or as good as everyone insists, you must have some taste, some experience of that. Otherwise, it's simply nothing more than a nice fantasy and may or may not be true.

The continuous gain of proof is irrefutable feedback that you can do it.

Change Comes First, Then Meaning

Change the way you look at things and the things you look at will change.
~ Wayne Dwyer

Understanding does not lead to change. Change leads to understanding. This does not mean logic, knowledge, and understanding don't come into the equation at all and don't have a place, because they do, but I want to offer to you the notion that, that place is later. Later, they are fun and interesting. Later, they can help to sustain the changes by helping you become aware of and actively pursue what you do want in life.

Right now, an ED is irrational thoughts, not just behaviours, and no amount of reasoning to do a "healthier" behaviour is going to create real change, because the moment you hit stress or overwhelm, your logic and willpower go out the window.

When fear is the captain of the ship, you'll revert back to ED behaviours without ever having had any say in it, let alone understand why. When you understand this, it is all so much simpler to understand why it is not your fault that logic and willpower have thus far failed to produce anything more than transient change.

Giving not Taking

No one is incurable.

AN may stem from things like a genetic predisposition and traumatic life events, but that is not why it persists, and therefore, it is not a life sentence.

AN has become your unconscious (default or natural) way of being, and those actions are out of your control. Therefore, the only true treatment will be that which is generative, that which helps you develop new choices and increases your power, resourcefulness, and self-efficacy to respond in useful ways to those same things which once derailed you so that your actions are happily under your control.

Essentially, treatment should always be geared toward putting the control back into your hands through giving you choices, not taking them away.

The Creation of Choice

Recovery is the increasing creation of choice.

We, that is the collective we as humans, become more capable by adding alternative resources (for example, knowledge, behaviours, skills), not by limiting, decreasing, or inhibiting them.

Which is why disapproval, punishment, threats, and other forms of coercion which unfortunately dominate in the mainstream "treatment" of AN and serve to take away the person's ability to develop and choose new options has been failing these people and their family and loved ones.

If you are reliant on the outside world for your health, be this through mean or kind ways, what will you do when that punishment, threat, coercion, guilt, love, or support is no longer available? You will resort straight back to the AN behaviour, because that is what you know.

On the other hand, when you have choices, you do not need to be coerced, bribed, threatened, punished, or even supported and praised to do the "right" thing, because you will have an effective way of meeting your needs without harming yourself or anyone else, naturally.

Speed It Up

No problem can be solved from the same level of consciousness that created it.
~Albert Einstein

I want you to get to where you want to be as soon as possible, and I want you to know that there are options out there to help you do this. Options which you may not have considered yet.

Recently, I spoke at the Australian Hypnotherapist Association Symposium, and at the close of the day, the last hour was devoted to questions directed at the speakers from the day. The last question asked of all of us was, "Where would you like to see the profession of hypnotherapy in ten years time?"

The answers were varied, but mine was simply that I'd like to see it offered as an option. I'd like to see it as something that is given as a choice or an option to people who are struggling to make changes in their lives. Alongside the options for psychology, psychiatry, and dietetics that we are presented with. I'd like that to happen far sooner than ten years, but however long it takes, I would love to see it happen.

This world is amazing, and the life you can live is incredible, and any time you waste in fear and not living it is a monumental loss.

There's also no forgetting that malnutrition is serious and AN, bulimia nervosa, and all eating disorders kill. Get intentional and deliberate help, help with a purpose, and most of all help not for the sake of help but help as a means to an end.

Hypnosis and NLP are means by which we can deliberately bring about real change. Which, in recovery from an eating disorder, is exactly what you want.

3. Life Coach

Why A Coach?

> *You cannot educate yourself to health and happiness. Health and happiness are experienced only in the doing.*
> *~ Bonnie Killip*

Since the 70s, coaching has gained immense popularity, and while the word has become a little tainted now, the truth is coaching is popular because it is proactive, and when done well, it works.

Coaching is about establishing goals and a direction you wish to head and then planning and taking the logical steps to get you there.

Working with a skilled coach allows you to get clear on what it is you want, bring what you want into full fruition, and continue moving forward.

Anorexia is Insidious

> *You don't have to see the whole staircase. Just take the first step.*

~ Martin Luther King

Anorexia is insidious. I know it is.

I know you can't truly be present or fully engaged with those things you want to be or with those you love because it is there. It is always there.

AN does not just affect what you eat. It affects your mood, focus, thoughts, attention, motivation, emotions, behaviours, relationships, work, friendships, finances and spirit.

Living with AN, you are in a strange pain twenty-four/seven, ranging from low level anxiety to full-blown, inconsolable sadness, panic, or rage.

AN is all-consuming, and as much as you wish it wasn't, AN is your life.

To be free of this is possible, and we've talked about how it is possible and the steps to take to make it more likely, but as we've also acknowledged, the recovery process is complicated by the fact that no part of your life has been left unaffected.

The reality is that when you recover, it is unlikely you are recovering immediately into the life you want.

There is likely still much to be addressed, learnt, and built upon until you are fully healthy and functioning at the level you desire and living the quality of life you desire.

Rather than be overwhelmed by how much you want to do or the big gap between where you are and where you want to be and never do any of it, consider seeking help from a professional coach and having the guidance on how to do it step by step while you're doing it.

Life is about enjoying the growing, the learning, and the expanding as much as it is about the attainment of goals.

The Defining Point in Which Your Life Changes is Now (Or Not)

> *You only live once, but if you do it right, once is enough.*
> *~ Mae West*

When you begin to move beyond starvation, the world opens. This can be a moment for overwhelm and retreat, or it can be the defining point in which your life changes; forever.

When the things which were once only ever hopes and dreams to you become actual choices you can make, you will benefit from having someone trained in coaching as part of your team.

Your life during and after recovery is, for the first time, yours, and you will have decisions to make depending on your interests, passions, and purpose.

It is a coach who can help you get clear on your direction, provide support, guidance, and challenge you in all the right ways in helping you reach your goals and live your passions and purpose. It is a coach that can help you function and live at your best.

Make Your Possibilities Manifest

> *You miss one hundred percent of the shots you don't take.*
> *~ Wayne Gretzky*

A skilled coach will help you make your possibilities reality. A great coach is not there to reassure you, make you feel better, or convince you that you are amazing, or even to tell you what to do. A great coach will not prescribe. A great coach will help you trust yourself, and they will help you to recognise and act in accordance with your values. A great coach will help you find the answers within yourself. A great coach knows they are there not to fix you but to help you grow.

A Coach Will Take You Out of Your Comfort Zone

> *I attribute my success to this: I never gave or took any excuses.*

~ Florence Nightingale

A great coach will push you where others in your life may stagnate or restrict your growth, capabilities, and achievements with their well-meaning desire to keep you safe and comfortable.

A great coach will help you become a better person, help you become the person you want to be and reach success in your chosen area/s far quicker than if you were to go it alone.

How far you take it is your choice, because a coach uses a specific set of professional skills to empower you, and it's not them doing the steps that will make your life exceptional, it is you.

They will walk you through each transition, and you will grow more than you ever imagined possible, but it is all your doing.

Summary to Recruiting Your Power Team

Life would be tragic if it weren't funny.
~ Steven Hawking

In summary, the people or person I suggest you recruit as your core Recovery Power Team are/is:

1. A Dietitian who specifically works with people in recovery from EDs.
2. An NLP and Clinical Hypnotherapy Practitioner
3. A Professional Life Coach

What Matters Most When Choosing Help

You can't be what you can't see.
~ Marian Wright Edelman

I've given specific titles and credentials of the people I would recommend for your recovery team because, clearly, qualifications matter in healthcare.

The fact that people have credentials means they've dedicated years of their lives and likely invested thousands of dollars into their education, and this is a good indicator that they not only have the knowledge but that they also have a passion for helping others. Therefore, these people are always your best place to start, but while these credentials are necessary, they alone do not mean someone can offer you what you need.

We are all unique in what we need, and the techniques of any therapy are limited by the therapist's ability to adapt them to meet your needs. There is no one method that will cure all people, not from EDs nor any other mental illness.

What I learnt during both my university degrees was invaluable, and I wholeheartedly recognise that I wouldn't be able to offer the level of help I do had I not become an expert in human function, health, and nutrition, because no matter how much effort you put in, if it is based off the wrong information, it is not going to get the right results.

Yet my biggest message regarding choosing those who can help you has less to do with the qualifications, credentials, or titles they go by and everything to do with the value they can add to your recovery. These are not the same.

Choosing your recovery team is about what they bring to your life.

At the end of the day, people are people, no matter what letters they have before or after their name, and this means they can only help to their level of understanding.

Chose the people that feel right to you.

Your experience may be completely different to mine.

Perhaps there were doctors, psychologists, and psychiatrists out there that could have helped me, I simply didn't find them.

I eventually found what worked for me, and so did anyone else who has recovered from an ED, and this is what you must do now.

You must find what works for you.

With all this in mind, there are three characteristics I believe are important when choosing your Recovery Power Team, no matter what credentials or titles they go by and I've listen them below.

The Three Most Important Characteristics of Your Chosen Recovery Team

> *What a teacher is, is more important than what he teaches.*
> *~ Karl Menninger*

1. Trust (You must believe they can help you).
    - Above all, they must believe in your ability to recover.
    - There will be a congruency between their personal and professional life (i.e., what they practice is what they preach).
    - They will always treat you with respect (which does not mean that they will not challenge you nor that you will be comfortable a hundred percent of the time, but it does mean they will not belittle, shame, or downplay your pain in disrespectful or dismissive ways).
2. Competence (Formally educated).
    - They must be able to give you the right information and education, especially with regard to your nutritional needs, because no matter how well-meaning or how long or how hard you persist, if the nutritional advice (or other advice) is incorrect, it's not going to get you the outcome you want.
3. Goal and Future Focused (Life Coaching skills)
    - They have a clear plan for getting you from where you are to where you want to be.

- Your "treatment" is less focussed on preventing worsening of your condition or in fleshing out past trauma but instead on how to get you from where you are to where you want to be.
- They competently run sessions, which are outcome focussed, and you are constantly and consistently developing the necessary skills, internally and externally, to reach your goals.

There you have it, my specific recommendations as to who you need on your Recovery Power Team. Whether you choose to take these suggestions or not is your choice.

I went through it all, and I'd really have loved some clear guidelines on how to recover fifteen years earlier than I found it. Who knows what my life would have been if I had, and who knows what your life can be from now.

Additional Support to Your Recovery Power Team

The purpose of our lives is to be happy.
~ Dalai Lama

From this core team or person, spread out and include as many layers of support as you desire. Reach out to those who are close to you. Allow your treatment to be something which can be discussed rather than something shameful and hidden.

Consider going to recovery groups or contacting others who are in recovery or have recovered, because they have so much to offer you.

However, always understand the difference between those who care and those who care and can help. Many may offer or want to help, fewer have the knowledge, skills, experience, and formal education to be able to be of the best help. Those who care can temporarily lessen your pain, but comfort is not cure.

You must get uncomfortable in recovery, at least for a time.

4.3 Environment

Control your destiny, or someone else will.
~ Jack Welch

I have deliberately left the topic of environment until last because I have wanted more than anything else to emphasise the power you have over your recovery. When all is said and done, your healing and a life of health can only ever come from you, and developing a strong sense of self will make you unstoppable.

However, there is the reality that the environment in which you live, including the people you interact with, has an enormous impact on you.

Therefore, it is important to not only heal yourself but also address areas in your life that may be keeping you stuck or hindering the life you want. If there are other barriers to your health, happiness, and living a successful life after AN, it is during your recovery and with the help of your treatment team that these should be addressed.

This can be tougher than it first sounds, because it may mean letting go of people, moving, or changing jobs or degree. All very real-life, hard things to do, even when you know they're the right thing to do.

4.4 Into the World: Practice

Be the change you wish to see in the world.
~ Mahatma Gandhi

Practice is the final step of the change process, because practice is what gives you the chance to change, and the chance to change is a chance at a different life.

Practice Doesn't Make Perfect

> *Progress is more important than perfection.*
> *~ Simon Sinek.*

Practice doesn't make perfect, and that is fantastic, because you are no longer aiming for perfection. Perfectionism inhibits life and inhibits greatness.

Practice makes a life.

Living A Good Life Does Not Come Through Any Other Means Than Living a Good Life.

> *The things that are easy to do are also easy not to do, that's the difference between success and failure.*
> *~ Jim Rohn*

When you can choose freely to think, feel, and behave in ways that are in line with your values, then you are practicing the life you want, and the reality is that practicing the life you want is indistinguishable from living the life you want.

Remember, at some stage, recovery becomes recovered.

Conclusion to *Ready, Now*

Courage is what we summon in the face of fear.
Love is what arises in the absence of fear.
~ Adyashanti

There are some hard experiences, truths, realisations, and discoveries that you will go through along the path of recovery. Many of which I have attempted to include in this book and many more I have not because, ultimately, your journey is your journey, and as such, it will be wholly and completely unique to you.

I, nor anyone else, can fully prepare you for what you are about to enter, and that is okay because that is what makes the journey yours.

Recovery is Creating You

Forgive yourself, develop yourself, be yourself, choose yourself, appreciate yourself, celebrate yourself, share your successes, share your heart, live your passions and purpose and never stop growing.
~ Bonnie Killip

Recovery need not always be focused on the pain and the fight, because the reality is, while it is hard, and this cannot be avoided, what it also is is sensational.

Recovery amidst the pain is a genuine opportunity of a lifetime.

Your experience with AN has contributed to who you are as a person today, but it has not, does not, and will never define you.

Although I would never choose to go through what I experienced again, I would also not erase it, even if I was given that option, because it forced me to see the world in a different way. Living with AN gave me the opportunity to learn skills I might otherwise have gone a lifetime without learning.

I rebuilt my body, and, most of all, I created my mind. I proved to myself the impossible.

My life with AN, and more importantly what I learnt to overcome this, no matter how unfair, helped me to develop my appreciation, reverence, and devotion to advancing wellbeing for all. That was the path my life took to reach the level it has, and for that, I have abundant appreciation.

It's About So Much More

World peace begins with inner peace.
~ Dalai Lama

As much as this book is about recovery from AN, it is about so much more. It is about recognising and creating a higher quality of life for all people.

My life is dedicated to advancing health, happiness, and wellbeing for all, not just those in recovery from EDs.

Mental illnesses have been on the rise for many years, and our efforts to combat and destroy them have largely been futile. In my opinion, a part of this is because we have so intensely focused on the illnesses and towards fighting. Where we must now shift our focus is toward what humans require in order to live happily, full and healthy lives, and then create more of that.

We need to focus on adding safety, meaning, connection, passion, and purpose to our lives in order to truly heal from and even prevent many of these illnesses.

We don't need more technology, more information, more data, more scientific advances, or some breakthrough to change the quality of our lives now. Of course, these advancements will come, and we will continue to increase our understanding of human health and illness, and these advancements will be fantastic and useful, but they are not necessary to live higher quality lives now.

We have all the resources and knowledge we need right now to make the world a safe and loving place for all.

We

The people who are crazy enough to think they can change the world are the ones who do.
~ Steve Jobs

With the tools, knowledge, and resources we have today, right now in this moment as you read these words, there is no need for so many people to live in fear, illness, and loneliness. There is no need for the huge level of human suffering which exists, not even the devastating world hunger and countries experiencing high levels of morbidity and mortality due to malnutrition, starvation, and unhygienic living conditions. There simply needs to be greater care, or perhaps even the level of care there is now combined with a greater coordination of the distribution of resources.

That's it. It really is that simple.

Imagine what we as individuals and as a society could achieve if we felt safe, loved, and connected?

Be the Person You Needed

Our deepest fear is not that we are inadequate. Our deepest fear is that we are powerful beyond measure. It is our light, not our darkness, that most frightens us. We ask ourselves, 'Who am I to be brilliant, gorgeous, talented, fabulous?' Actually, who are you not to be? You are a child of God. Your playing small does not serve the world. There is nothing enlightened about shrinking so that other people won't feel insecure around you. We are all meant to shine, as children do. We were born to make manifest the glory of God that is within us. It's not just in some of us; it's in everyone. And as we let our own light shine, we unconsciously give other people permission to do the same. As we are liberated from our own fear, our presence automatically liberates others." ~ Marianne Williamson

What would you need to do to become the person who could have stopped you from ever becoming sick or the person who could have helped you heal long ago?

Take care of yourself and live what's possible, not just for you but for the world.

No one is asking for the perfect record from you, just your authenticity.

Don't Do It

To be yourself in a world that is constantly trying to make you something else is the greatest accomplishment.
~ Ralph Waldo Emerson

You don't have to act on this information just yet.

In fact, you never have to act on any of the information or advice in this book or that I or anyone else gives you in life if it is not in alignment with your values.

If I ever suggest some advice or information that does not fit with your values, simply don't take it.

I am not here to tell you right or wrong.

I am not here to convince you to do x, y, or z.

I am not here to tell you how to live your life nor to beg you to change. I am not even here to convince you or argue with you that you should recover. I am here to help you see that there are other possibilities for how you can live. I am here to show you there are other possibilities for how you can experience the rest of your life.

Whether you choose any of these options or not is not up to me nor anyone else but you. It is up to you.

5.1 Parting Words

When you want something all the universe conspires in helping you to achieve it.
~ Paulo Coelho

As my parting words, I want to say that there is nothing etherical, nothing saintly, and nothing romantic about anorexia.

AN doesn't make you special. You are not brave or more deserving because you struggle and achieve through the pain. Tolerating and enduring the abuse of AN does not make you strong or valiant.

You are not protecting anyone or making anyone else's life easier by denying, hiding, or pushing though. It takes much more courage to choose yourself.

It takes much more courage to choose recovery, and recovery is the only way you will experience freedom and the only way you will ever truly help and connect with those you love and those you are yet to love.

The beliefs that recovery is easier the sooner you do it and if you leave it too late you have less chance of recovering and that recovery requires a lengthy healing period are misconceptions. Your recovery is dependent only on what you choose to do in this moment and the next moment and the moment after that, and this is entirely independent on

Ready Now

what has happened to you and what you have been capable of or what you have done in the past.

There is no beautiful secret that AN has yet to reveal to you if only you persist a little longer. You know it all.

Use where you are now as a leaping board to where you want to be.

Your Turn

After reading this compilation of words I've sewn together into a curious tapestry of knowledge over the past almost eight years since my recovery, there is just one final question I want to offer you.

One final question for you to take away and ask yourself and know with all your heart that your answer is the most important answer you will ever give because it will determine the course of the rest of your life.

It's a very simple question and the it is…

What are you going to do with all this knowledge you now have?

Yours in health, happiness, and fulfillment, always,
~Bonnie

Reference

1. Steinglass J, Sysko R, Mayer L, Berner L, Schebendach J, Wang Y, Chen H, Albano A, Simpson H, Walsh B. Pre-meal anxiety and food intake in anorexia nervosa. Appetite. 2010;55(2):214–218.
2. 3001. Kaye W, Fudge J, Paulus M. New insight into symptoms and neurocircuit function of anorexia nervosa. Nat Rev Neurosci. 2009;10(8):573–584.
3. 36. Bulik C, Sullivan PF, Tozzi F, Furberg H, Lichtenstein P, Pedersen NL. Prevalence, heritability and prospective risk factors for anorexia nervosa. Arch Gen Psychiatry. 2006;63(3):305–12.
4. Nunn K, Frampton I, Fuglet TS, Torzsok-Sonnevend M, Lask B. Anorexia nervosa and the insula. Medical Hypotheses. Mar 2011: 76(3);353-357.
5. Bulik CM, Sullivan PF, Tozzi F, Furberg H, Lichtenstein P, Pedersen NL. Prevalence, Heritability, and Prospective Risk Factors for Anorexia Nervosa. Arch Gen Psychiatry. 2006;63(3):305–312.
6. Strober M, Freeman R, Lampert C, Diamond J, Kaye W. Controlled Family Study of Anorexia Nervosa and Bulimia Nervosa: Evidence of Shared Liability and Transmission of Partial Syndromes. The Am J of Psych. 1 Mar 2000: 157(3);393-401.
7. Yilmaz, Z., Hardaway, J. A. & Bulik, C. M. Genetics and epigenetics of eating disorders. Adv. Genomics Genet. 5, 131–150 (2015).
8. Bulik CM, Sullivan PF, Tozzi F, Furberg H, Lichtenstein P, Pedersen NL. Prevalence, heritability, and prospective risk factors for anorexia nervosa. Arch Gen Psychiatry. 2006 Mar; 63(3):305-12.
9. Klump KL, Miller KB, Keel PK, McGue M, Iacono WG. Genetic and environmental influences on anorexia nervosa syndromes in a population-based twin sample. Psychol Med. 2001 May; 31(4):737-40.
10. Kortegaard LS, Hoerder K, Joergensen J, Gillberg C, Kyvik KO. A preliminary population-based twin study of self-reported eating disorder. Psychol Med. 2001 Feb; 31(2):361-5.
11. Mazzeo SE, Mitchell KS, Bulik CM, Reichborn-Kjennerud T, Kendler KS, Neale MC. Assessing the heritability of anorexia nervosa symptoms using a marginal maximal likelihood approach. Psychol Med. 2009 Mar; 39(3):463-73.

12. Wade TD, Bulik CM, Neale M, Kendler KS. Anorexia nervosa and major depression: shared genetic and environmental risk factors. Am J Psychiatry. 2000 Mar; 157(3):469-71.
13. Hunna J. Watson, Zeynep Yilmaz, Laura M. Thornton, Christopher Hübel, Jonathan R. I. Coleman, Héléna A. Gaspar, Julien Bryois, Anke Hinney, Virpi M. Leppä, Manuel Mattheisen, Sarah E. Medland, Stephan Ripke, Shuyang Yao, Paola Giusti-Rodríguez, Ken B. Hanscombe, Kirstin L. Purves, Roger A. H. Adan, Lars Alfredsson, Tetsuya Ando, Ole A. Andreassen, Jessica H. Baker, Wade H. Berrettini, Ilka Boehm, Claudette Boni, Vesna Boraska Perica, Katharina Buehren, Roland Burghardt, Matteo Cassina, Sven Cichon, Maurizio Clementi, Roger D. Cone, Philippe Courtet, Scott Crow, James J. Crowley, Unna N. Danner, Oliver S. P. Davis, Martina de Zwaan, George Dedoussis, Daniela Degortes, Janiece E. DeSocio, Danielle M. Dick, Dimitris Dikeos, Christian Dina, Monika Dmitrzak-Weglarz, Elisa Docampo, Laramie E. Duncan, Karin Egberts, Stefan Ehrlich, Geòrgia Escaramís, Tõnu Esko, Xavier Estivill, Anne Farmer, Angela Favaro, Fernando Fernández-Aranda, Manfred M. Fichter, Krista Fischer, Manuel Föcker, Lenka Foretova, Andreas J. Forstner, Monica Forzan, Christopher S. Franklin, Steven Gallinger, Ina Giegling, Johanna Giuranna, Fragiskos Gonidakis, Philip Gorwood, Monica Gratacos Mayora, Sébastien Guillaume, Yiran Guo, Hakon Hakonarson, Konstantinos Hatzikotoulas, Joanna Hauser, Johannes Hebebrand, Sietske G. Helder, Stefan Herms, Beate Herpertz-Dahlmann, Wolfgang Herzog, Laura M. Huckins, James I. Hudson, Hartmut Imgart, Hidetoshi Inoko, Vladimir Janout, Susana Jiménez-Murcia, Antonio Julià, Gursharan Kalsi, Deborah Kaminská, Jaakko Kaprio, Leila Karhunen, Andreas Karwautz, Martien J. H. Kas, James L. Kennedy, Anna Keski-Rahkonen, Kirsty Kiezebrink, Youl-Ri Kim, Lars Klareskog, Kelly L. Klump, Gun Peggy S. Knudsen, Maria C. La Via, Stephanie Le Hellard, Robert D. Levitan, Dong Li, Lisa Lilenfeld, Bochao Danae Lin, Jolanta Lissowska, Jurjen Luykx, Pierre J. Magistretti, Mario Maj, Katrin Mannik, Sara Marsal, Christian R. Marshall, Morten Mattingsdal, Sara McDevitt, Peter McGuffin, Andres Metspalu, Ingrid Meulenbelt, Nadia Micali, Karen Mitchell, Alessio Maria Monteleone, Palmiero Monteleone, Melissa A. Munn-Chernoff, Benedetta Nacmias, Marie Navratilova, Ioanna Ntalla, Julie K. O'Toole, Roel A. Ophoff, Leonid Padyukov, Aarno Palotie, Jacques Pantel, Hana Papezova, Dalila Pinto, Raquel Rabionet, Anu Raevuori, Nicolas Ramoz, Ted Reichborn-Kjennerud, Valdo Ricca, Samuli Ripatti, Franziska Ritschel, Marion Roberts, Alessandro Rotondo, Dan Rujescu, Filip Rybakowski, Paolo Santonastaso, André Scherag, Stephen W. Scherer, Ulrike Schmidt, Nicholas J. Schork, Alexandra Schosser, Jochen Seitz, Lenka Slachtova, P. Eline Slagboom, Margarita C. T. Slof-Op 't Landt, Agnieszka Slopien, Sandro Sorbi, Beata Świątkowska, Jin P. Szatkiewicz, Ioanna Tachmazidou, Elena Tenconi, Alfonso Tortorella, Federica Tozzi, Janet Treasure, Artemis Tsitsika, Marta Tyszkiewicz-Nwafor, Konstantinos Tziouvas, Annemarie A. van Elburg, Eric F. van Furth, Gudrun Wagner, Esther Walton, Elisabeth Widen,

Eleftheria Zeggini, Stephanie Zerwas, Stephan Zipfel, Andrew W. Bergen, Joseph M. Boden, Harry Brandt, Steven Crawford, Katherine A. Halmi, L. John Horwood, Craig Johnson, Allan S. Kaplan, Walter H. Kaye, James E. Mitchell, Catherine M. Olsen, John F. Pearson, Nancy L. Pedersen, Michael Strober, Thomas Werge, David C. Whiteman, D. Blake Woodside, Garret D. Stuber, Scott Gordon, Jakob Grove, Anjali K. Henders, Anders Juréus, Katherine M. Kirk, Janne T. Larsen, Richard Parker, Liselotte Petersen, Jennifer Jordan, Martin Kennedy, Grant W. Montgomery, Tracey D. Wade, Andreas Birgegård, Paul Lichtenstein, Claes Norring, Mikael Landén, Nicholas G. Martin, Preben Bo Mortensen, Patrick F. Sullivan, Gerome Breen, Cynthia M. Bulik. Genome-wide association study identifies eight risk loci and implicates metabo-psychiatric origins for anorexia nervosa. Nature Genetics, 2019.
14. Devlin B, Bacanu SA, Klump KL, Bulik CM, Fichter MM, Halmi KA, Kaplan AS, Strober M, Treasure J, Woodside DB, Berrettini WH, Kaye WH. Linkage analysis of anorexia nervosa incorporating behavioural covariates. Human Molecular Genetics. 15 March 2002: 11(6):689–696.
15. Kaye WH, Klump KL, Frank GKW, Strober M. Anorexia and Bulimia Nervosa. Annual Review of Medicine. Feb 2000: 51(1); 299-313.
16. Wade T, Martin NG, Tiggemann M. Genetic and environmental risk factors for the weight and shape concerns characteristic of bulimia nervosa. Psychol Med. 1998 Jul; 28(4):761-71
17. Slade P. Towards a functional analysis of anorexia nervosa and bulimia nervosa. British Journal of Clinical Psychology. 1982. 21: 167-179.
18. Hill L, Peck SK, Wierenga CE and Kaye WH. Applying neurobiology to the treatment of adults with anorexia nervosa. Journal of Eating Disorders. 2016. 4:31.
19. Meczekalski B, Podfigurna-Stopa A, Katulski K. Long-term consequences of anorexia nervosa. Maturitas. 2013. 75;215-220.
20. Ihab Lamzabi, Sahr Syed, Vijaya B. Reddy, Richa Jain, Aparna Harbhajanka, Ponni Arunkumar; Myocardial Changes in a Patient With Anorexia Nervosa: A Case Report and Review of Literature, American Journal of Clinical Pathology. 1 May 2015. 143(5):734–737.
21. Casiero D, Frishman WH. Cardiovascular complications of eating disorders. Cardiol Rev. 2006. 14:227-231.
22. Rose M, Greene RM. Cardiovascular complications during prolonged starvation. West J Med. 1979. 130:170.
23. Olivares JL, Vazquez M, Fleta J et al. Cardiac findings in adolescents with anorexia nervosa at diagnosis and after weight restoration. Eur J Pediatr. 2005. 164:383.
24. de Simone G, Scalfi L, Galderisi M et al. Cardiac abnormalities in young women with anorexia nervosa. Br Heart J. 1994. 71:287.
25. Harris EC, Barraclough B (1998) Excess mortality of mental disorder. Br J Psychiatry 173: 11–53.

26. Sachs KV, Harnke B, Mehler PS, Krantz MJ. Cardiovascular complications of anorexia nervosa: A systematic review. Int J Eat Disord. 2016 Mar: 46(3); 238-48.
27. Otto B, Cuntz U, Fruehauf E et al. Weight gain decreases elevated plasma ghrelin concentrations of patients with anorexia nervosa. Eur. J. Endocrinol. 2001. 145(5), 669-673.
28. Laessle RG, Fischer MMM, Fishter K, Pirke M, Krieg JC. Cortisol levels and vigilance in eating disorder patients. Psychoneuroendocrinology. 17, 5, 1992, 475-484.
29. Hamsher K, Halmi KA, & Benton AL. Prediction of outcome in anorexia nervosa from neuropsychological status. Psychiatry Research, 1981. 4, 79-88.
30. Katzman, D K, Christensen, B, Young, A R, & Zipursky, R B. Starving the brain: Structural abnormalities and cognitive impairment in adolescents with anorexia nervosa. Seminars in Clinical Neuropsychiatry. 2001. 6, 146-152.
31. Tchanturia, Kate; Anderluh, Marija BRECELJ; Morris, Robin G; Rabe-hesketh, Sophia; Collier, David A; et al. Cognitive flexibility in anorexia nervosa and bulimia nervosa. Journal of the International Neuropsychological Society: JINS; Cambridge. 2014.10:4); 513-20.
32. Kingston, K, Szmukler, G, Andrewers, B, Tress, B, & Desmond, P. Neuropsychological and structural brain changes in anorexia nervosa before and after refeeding. Psychological Medicine. 1996. 26, 15-28.
33. Lauer, C J, Gorzewski, B, Gerlinghoff, M, Backmund, H, & Zihl, J. Neuropsychological assessments before and after treatment in patients with anorexia nervosa and bulimia nervosa. Journal of Psychiatric Research. 1999. 33, 129-138.
34. Pendleton Jones, B, Duncan, C, Brouwers, P, & Mirsky, A. Cognition in eating disorders. Journal of Clinical and Experimental Neuropsychology. 1991. 13, 711-728.
35. Lena SM, Fiocco AJ, Leyenaar JK. The role of cognitive deficits in the development of eating disorders. Neuropsychology Review. 2004. 14, 99–113.
36. Southgate L, Tchanturia K, Treasure J (2009). Neuropsychology in eating disorders. In The Neuropsychology of Mental Illness (ed. S. J. Wood, N. B. Allen and C. Pantelis), pp. 316–325. Cambridge University Press: Cambridge.
37. Oberndorfer T, Kaye W, Simmons A, Strigo I, Matthews S. Demand-specific alteration of medial prefrontal cortex response during an ihhibition task in recovered anorexic women. Int J Eat Disord. 2011;44(1):1–8.
38. Lock J, Garrett A, Beenhakker J, Reiss A. Aberrant brain activation during a response inhibition task in adolescent eating disorder subtypes. Am J Psychiatry. 2011;168(1):55–64.
39. Zastrow A, Kaiser S, Stippich C, Walthe S, Herzog W, Tchanturia K, Belger A, Weisbrod M, Treasure J, Friederich H. Neural correlates of impaired cognitive-behavioral flexibility in anorexia nervosa. Am J Psychiatry. 2009;166(5):608–16.

40. Wierenga C, Bischoff-Grethe A, Melrose A, Grenesko-Stevens E, Irvine Z, Wagner A, Simmons A, Matthews S, Yau W-Y, Finneman-Notestine C, Kaye W. Altered BOLD response during inhibitory and error processing in adolescents with anorexi anervosa. PLoS One. 2014;9:392017.
41. King JA, Frank GKW, Thompson PM, Ehrlich S. Structural neuroimaging of anorexia nervosa: Future directions in the quest for mechanisms underlying dynamic alterations. Biol Psychiatry. 2018: 83;224-234.
42. King JA, Geisler D, Ritschel F, Boehm I, Seidel M, Roschinski B, et al. Global cortical thinning in acute anorexia nervosa normalizes following long-term weight restoration. Biol Psychiatry. 2015: 77;624-632
43. Titova OE, Hjorth OC, Schiöth HB, Brooks SJ. Anorexia nervosa is linked to reduced brain structure in reward and somatosensory regions: A meta-analysis of VBM studies. BMC Psychiatry. 2013: 13;110.
44. Seitz J, Bühren K, von Polier GG, Heussen N, Herpertz-Dahlmann B, Konrad K. Morphological changes in the brain of acutely ill and weight-recovered patients with anorexia nervosa. A meta-analysis and qualitative review. Z Kinder Jugendpsychiatrie Psychother. 2014: 42;7-17.
45. Bernardoni F, King JA, Geisler D, Birkenstock J, Tam FI, Weidner K, Roessner V, White T, Ehrlich S Nutritional Status Affects Cortical Folding: Lessons Learned From Anorexia Nerv osa. Biol Psychiatry. 2018 Nov 1;84(9):692-701.
46. Youl-RiKim[a]Chan-HyungKim[b]ValentinaCardi[c]Jin-SupEom[d]YooriSeong[a]JanetTreasure[c] Intranasal oxytocin attenuates attentional bias for eating and fat shape stimuli in patients with anorexia nervosa. Psychoneuroendocrinology. 2014. 44; 133-142.
47. Derman O, Kiliç EZ. Edema can be a handicap in treatment of anorexia nervosa. Turk J Pediatr. 2009; 51(6):593-7.
48. Brown JM, Mehler PS, Harris RH. Medical complications occurring in adolescents with anorexia nervosa. West J Med 2000;172:189–93.
49. Woodside DB. A review of anorexia nervosa and bulimia nervosa. Curr Probl Pediatr 1995;25(2):67–89.
50. Beumont PJ, Russell JD, Touyz SW. Treatment of anorexia nervosa. Lancet 1993;341(8861):1635–40.
51. Carney CP, Andersen AE. Eating disorders. Guide to medical evaluation and complications. Psychiatr Clin North Am 1996;19:657–79.
52. Assadi SN. What are the effects of psychological stress and physical work on blood lipid profiles?. Medicine (Baltimore). 2017;96(18):e6816.
53. RigaudD, TallonneauI, VergèsB. Hypercholesterolaemia in anorexia nervosa: frequency and changes during refeeding. Diabetes Metab. 2009;35:57–63.
54. OhwadaR, HottaM, OikawaS, TakanoK. Etiology of hypercholesterolemia in patients with anorexia nervosa. Int J Eat Disord. 2006;39:598–60

55. MatzkinVB, GeisslerC, ConiglioR, SellesJ, BelloM. Cholesterol concentrations in patients with anorexia nervosa and in healthy controls. Int J Psychiatr Nurs Res. 2006;11:1283–93.
56. Bluemel S, Menne D, Milos G, Goetze O, Fried M, Schwizer W, et al. Relationship of body weight with gastrointestinal motor and sensory function: studies in anorexia nervosa and obesity. BMC Gastroenterology 2017;17.
57. Kerr KL, Moseman SE, Avery JA, Bodurka J, Zucker NL, Simmons WK. Altered Insula Activity during Visceral Interoception in Weight-Restored Patients with Anorexia Nervosa. Neuropsychopharmacology 2016 01;41(2):521-528.
58. Scalfi L, Polito A, Bianchi L, Marra M, al e. Body composition changes in patients with anorexia nervosa after complete weight recovery. Eur J Clin Nutr 2002 01;56(1):15-20.
59. Hatch A, Madden S, Kohn M, et al. (2010) Anorexia nervosa: Towards an integrative neuroscience model. European Eating Disorders Review 18: 165–179.
60. Friederich H, Walther S, Bendszus M, Biller A, Thomann P, Zeigermann S, et al. Grey matter abnormalities within cortico-limbic-striatal circuits in acute and weight-restored anorexia nervosa patients. Neuroimage 2012 Jan 16;59(2):1106-1113.
61. Kohn MR, Madden S and Clarke SD. Refeeding in anorexia nervosa: Increased safety and efficiency through understanding the pathophysiology of protein calorie malnutrition. Current Opinion in Pediatrics. 2011. 23: 390–394.
62. Marrazzi MA, Luby ED. An auto-addiction opioid model of chronic anorexia nervosa. Int J Eat Disord. 1986;5:191-208.
63. Heubner HF. Endorphins, Eating Disorders and other Addictive Behaviours. New York. W. W. Norton 1993.
64. Barron, Leanne J; Barron, Robert F; Johnson, Jeremy C S; Wagner, Ingrid; Ward, Cameron J B; et al. A retrospective analysis of biochemical and haematological parameters in patients with eating disorders. Journal of Eating Disorders; London. 2017. Vol. 5.

www.ingramcontent.com/pod-product-compliance
Lightning Source LLC
Chambersburg PA
CBHW052137070526
44585CB00017B/1863